The Painless Guide to Mastering Clinical Acid-Base

Benjamin Abelow, M.D.

The Painless Guide to Mastering Clinical Acid-Base
Copyright © 2016 Benjamin Abelow, M.D. All rights reserved.

ISBN: 13:978-1517438029
ISBN: 10:1517438020

This book is dedicated in loving memory to my mother,
Phoebe Meyerowitz Abelow, and father,
Irving Abelow, M.D.

Table of Contents

Acknowledgments

Peter Aronson, M.D., Professor of Internal Medicine and of Cellular and Molecular Physiology, and previously Chief of the Section of Nephrology at Yale University School of Medicine, taught me acid-base when I was a student and has remained a valued teacher and adviser ever since. At the inception of this project, Peter helped me refine my vision for this book and, as work progressed, he read and commented thoughtfully on two different drafts of the manuscript.

Linda Pellico, Ph.D., A.P.R.N., critical care specialist and Associate Professor at Yale University School of Nursing, welcomed me into her classes as a guest lecturer when I was teaching at Yale. Linda thoroughly critiqued an early draft of the manuscript, providing a variety of comments and suggestions that substantially improved the quality and usability of the text.

Steven Coca, M.D., Assistant Professor of Medicine (nephrology) at Yale University School of Medicine, read and commented on a late draft of the manuscript and generously discussed a wide variety of substantive and pedagogical issues with me. Steve's clinical expertise and uncommon good sense were truly invaluable.

For over a decade, Nicolaos E. Madias, M.D., the Maurice S. Segal, M.D. Professor of Medicine at Tufts University School of Medicine and Chair of the Department of Medicine at St. Elizabeth's Medical Center, has graciously encouraged my efforts to explain acid-base to a non-specialist audience. For this book, Nick read a late draft, provided suggestions and corrections, and offered a generous endorsement.

Additional help came from many quarters. Scott Beegle, M.D., critiqued a draft of the respiratory chapters, and Julian L. Seifter, M.D., shared his expertise about several vexed topics. Jack Hammer, Ph.D, reviewed early drafts of the chemistry material and brought to light a number of technical and pedagogical issues. John Hayden, B.S.E., and Jeanette Wasserstein, Ph.D., provided encouragement and sage advice. I am grateful to Dr. Nancy Angoff for her support.

Alexandra Tinari, M.F.A., provided superb editing of concept, content, and copy. Pam Auerbach and Carolyn Friedman, F.N.P., were trusted strategic and editorial advisers. Mary, whose last name is a mystery, patiently guided me through the publishing process. My brother, Adam Abelow, who played a key role in my intellectual development by helping teach me to write clearly and logically, reviewed and commented on parts of the manuscript. Suzanne Rosencrans, J.D., was generous with her publishing advice. I also wish to acknowledge the important contributions of Drs. Fred Wright and Asghar Rastegar to my overall acid-base education.

Finally, almost two dozen medical and nursing students at Yale reviewed one or more complete drafts of the manuscript. Their extensive feedback and suggestions influenced every aspect of the book. In alphabetical order, I gratefully acknowledge Andre Alcon, Stephanie Andrade, Deepak Atri, Ani Bagdasarian, Willa Campbell, Nicholas Golinvaux, Abhijeet Gummadavelli, Jessie Zhe Hou, Olga Laur, Eleanor

Miller, Rachel Morse, Caitlin Paul, Joseph Patterson, Carolyn Perotti, Britt Sandler, Amanda Strauss, Colin Tominey, James Tooley, Samantha XY Wang, and Ke Zhang. I also thank Melissa Herrin, Sasha Deutsch-Link, and Nicholas Apostolopoulos for their suggestions.

In the course of writing two books on acid-base, I have come to see one of my most important authorial functions as that of medium: finding creative ways to access, integrate, and communicate the insights of many exceptional researchers, teachers, and learners. If this book proves of value, then each person listed above deserves a meaningful share of the credit. Responsibility for any shortcomings or errors is mine alone.

Introduction

Why read this book? After all, acid-base is covered in lectures, class notes, text chapters, and review books. Isn't it possible to piece the subject together for yourself? The sad fact is that, using currently available resources and teaching methods, most students and clinicians do not learn acid-base adequately. Ask any ten clinicians if they're comfortable with acid-base and you're likely to get more than a few sheepish looks.

Further, most students and clinicians ultimately recognize their deficit, and then spend a great deal of time, catch-as-catch-can, trying to repair their understanding. But because a solid foundation is lacking, simply trying to fill in the gaps does not fix the problem. As a result, many people end up with the worst of both worlds: inadequate knowledge and a great deal of wasted time. Along the way, patient care, which is the point of the whole endeavor, suffers immeasurably.

I wrote this book to provide a better way, one that lets you learn acid-base correctly right from the start. You'll master all the fundamentals. You'll learn the common causes of both simple and mixed acid-base disturbances, and their pathophysiology. You'll really understand blood gas interpretation and the anion gap, and you'll get in-depth, systematic experience solving diagnostic problems (see the carefully structured problem sequences, with detailed explanations, in Chapters 11, 12, and 13). Finally, you won't waste time on fruitless remediation. Rather, if you ever do choose to spend additional time on acid-base, your efforts will be truly productive, leading you towards exceptional expertise.

Like reading a chest x-ray and interpreting an EKG, understanding and diagnosing acid-base disorders is a core area of clinical knowledge. Taking the time to read this brief book now will benefit you—and your patients—throughout your career.

Good luck, and enjoy!

Benjamin Abelow, M.D.

P.S. If you have suggestions for future editions, or simply want to let me know what you think of the book, you can reach me at AcidBaseMadeClear@gmail.com. Please write "acid-base" in the subject line.

How To Make This Book Work for You

There are many ways you can use this book, depending on your needs and available time. Find one that works for you. Here are some ideas.

Cover to Cover. By reading cover to cover, you'll get an easy-to-read, private tutorial that will teach you acid-base from the ground up, culminating in a rich experience of diagnostic problem solving. In the opening chapters, you'll learn the fundamentals of acid-base chemistry and physiology. You'll then build on that foundation by learning pathophysiology, diagnosis, and treatment concepts.

Chemistry and Physiology. If your immediate goal is to learn acid-base chemistry and physiology, read Chapters 1–4. If you want to take the next step, and get a quick introduction to clinical acid-base, continue to Chapter 5. These early chapters make excellent stand-alone reading for medical students who are currently focusing on preclinical material.

Clinical Only. If you want a complete course in clinical acid-base and already know the fundamentals of acid-base chemistry and physiology, simply start at Chapter 5. If you need to solidify your understanding of the overall acid-base system, read Chapter 2 first.

Arterial Blood Gases. If you want to learn or review blood gas interpretation, read Chapter 5 followed by Chapter 11, working all problems as you go. Taken together, these two chapters form a brief but thorough course on blood gas interpretation. If you're shaky on basic terms and concepts, read Chapter 2 first.

Specific Topics. Each chapter is designed to stand alone as much as possible, so you can read selectively, according to your needs. Many sections within chapters are also self contained. Do you need to learn about lactic acidosis? Read pages 69–72. Want to learn about the anion gap? Read pages 140–147.

Boards & Certifying Exams. You can quickly learn or review a lot of test-relevant acid-base, with an emphasis on interpreting blood gases (a topic that is frequently tested), by following these six steps: (1) In the optional review (pp. 1–13), read only the boxes and the summary on the last page. (2) Read the chapter previews on pages vii–viii. (3) Read Chapter 2 in its entirety. (4) Starting with Chapter 1, go through each chapter in the book doing the following: read the first paragraph of the chapter, then read the summary on the final page, then page through the chapter from start to finish, studying just the figures, tables, and any small boxes (skip any large, page-size boxes you encounter). Some things won't make full sense to you out of context; that's normal, so don't worry about it; just get what you can and keep going! (5) Master blood gas interpretation by reading Chapters 5 and 11 from start to finish, working all problems. (6) Master the anion gap by reading pp. 140–147, working all problems.

Diagnosis. If you want to learn the full range of acid-base diagnosis and already have some background in acid-base pathophysiology, read Chapter 5 followed by Chapters 11 and 12, working all problems. Then read the brief sections on diagnostic tests on pages 80–84 and 100–102. Finally, work through Chapter 13.

A Note on Footnotes

This book contains optional footnotes designed to enrich your learning experience. Some offer extra help, clarify terms, or provide mnemonics. Others give clinical tie-ins or let you go deeper into a topic. Read those notes that fit your needs and interests, and feel free to skip the rest. The essentials are all in the text.

Chapter Previews

An Optional Review—From Atoms to Buffers

This book is written for a broad audience with varied pre-clinical backgrounds. If you haven't had a full-year college chemistry course, this review will get you off to a strong start.

1. The Chemical Foundation: The Bicarbonate Buffer System

Buffers help stabilize pH when acid or base loads are present. The bicarbonate buffer is the most important buffer in the body. It serves as the chemical foundation on which acid-base physiology, pathophysiology, and diagnosis are layered.

2. Overview of Acid-Base: A Balancing Act

This pivotal chapter explains how the body's pH is determined by the balance between plasma bicarbonate concentration, which is regulated by the kidney, and PCO_2, which is regulated by the lung. The chapter also introduces the four pairs of terms you must know to communicate clearly about acid-base.

3. Acid-Base Physiology: The Lung

This chapter explains how the lung regulates the PCO_2 of arterial blood, and it describes how this PCO_2 changes as the blood moves through the circulatory system. The chapter provides a strong foundation for studying the respiratory acid-base disturbances (respiratory acidosis and respiratory alkalosis).

4. Acid-Base Physiology: The Kidney

After a quick review of general kidney physiology, this chapter focuses on two key renal processes that regulate the plasma bicarbonate level: bicarbonate reabsorption and bicarbonate regeneration. This chapter provides an excellent foundation for studying the metabolic acid-base disturbances (metabolic acidosis and metabolic alkalosis).

5. Compensation: A "Damage Limitation" Strategy

When acid-base disturbances arise, compensation kicks in to help stabilize pH. The extent of compensation can be predicted using "rules of thumb." You'll work problems to see how these rules are applied. This chapter provides an essential foundation for interpreting blood gases.

6. Metabolic Acidosis

Metabolic acidosis is a pathologic process that reduces plasma bicarbonate concentration, which in turn lowers pH. This chapter explains the pathophysiology and clinical causes, including diarrhea, ketoacidosis, lactic acidosis, and kidney disease. The chapter also covers important diagnostic tests and treatment concepts.

7. Metabolic Alkalosis

Metabolic alkalosis is the opposite of metabolic acidosis. It is a pathologic process that raises plasma bicarbonate concentration, which in turn increases pH. This chapter explains the pathophysiology and clinical causes, including vomiting and diuretics. The chapter also covers important diagnostic tests and treatment concepts.

8. Respiratory Acidosis

Respiratory acidosis arises when the lung is unable to eliminate CO_2 normally, causing an increase in PCO_2, which in turn lowers pH. This chapter examines the underlying pathophysiology and the common clinical causes. The chapter also explains the load-strength model of respiratory acidosis and its application to treatment.

9. Respiratory Alkalosis

Respiratory alkalosis is the opposite of respiratory acidosis. Respiratory alkalosis occurs when the rate of ventilation is abnormally elevated, causing a decrease in PCO_2, which in turn raises pH. Respiratory alkalosis always indicates that the stimulus to breathe is abnormally increased. Understanding respiratory alkalosis can help you identify life-threatening conditions such as sepsis.

10. Mixed Disturbances

When two or more distinct acid-base abnormalities are present at the same time, a mixed disturbance is said to exist. By teaching you the most common clinical causes of mixed disturbances, this chapter helps you recognize mixed disturbances when you encounter them.

11. Diagnosis with Arterial Blood Gases

This hands-on chapter teaches you how to diagnose acid-base disturbances from the arterial blood gas. You'll work through a carefully structured sequence of practice problems, with full explanations, to build knowledge and confidence.

12. Diagnosis with Venous Bicarbonate, Anion Gap, and Potassium

Blood gases are not the only way to diagnose acid-base disturbances. Another invaluable tool is the set of routine "chemistries" done on a venous blood sample. Once again, you'll develop knowledge and confidence by working through a carefully structured sequence of practice problems.

13. All Together Now: Integrative Problems

This final chapter challenges you with twelve integrative diagnostic problems that build on all you've learned. These problems and their detailed solutions show you how far you've come, take your knowledge to the next level, and provide a bridge to working with patients in the clinical setting.

An Optional Review— From Atoms to Buffers

I've included this review for those readers who have not had the benefit of a full-year college chemistry course. If you fall into this category, reading this review will give you a solid foundation for the rest of the book. Don't worry about memorizing—just focus on meaning, so the ideas make sense as you read them. **Bolded** words and phrases tend to recur in subsequent chapters, so give those a bit of added attention. For emphasis, key points are repeated in the boxes. If you already have a good general chemistry background but nonetheless want a quick refresher, feel free to skim or read selectively.

Atoms, Molecules, and Ions

Matter is made of atoms. Some atoms exist alone, as single, freestanding atoms, but most exist in groups of two or more atoms bound together into a unified structure by chemical bonds. These multi-atom structures are called **molecules**. An example is **carbon dioxide (CO_2)**. Sometimes molecules are made of a single kind of atom. For example, **oxygen** usually exists as a pair of oxygen atoms bound together (O_2).

When an atom or molecule carries an electrical charge, it is called an **ion**. The charge on an ion can be either positive (+) or negative (–). Examples are **sodium (Na^+)**, **potassium (K^+)**[*], **chloride (Cl^-)**, and **bicarbonate (HCO_3^-)**. The ion's charge is indicated in the superscript. When the + or – sign does not have a number attached, as in the examples just given, the ion has a single charge (+1 or –1). Some ions carry two or more charges. **Calcium (Ca^{2+})** and **magnesium (Mg^{2+})** ions have a double positive charge.

An ion with a positive charge can be referred to by a general phrase like "positive ion" or by the specific term **cation**. An ion with a negative charge can be referred to by a general phrase like "negative ion" or by the specific term **anion**.[**] Chemical structures that have a carbon-hydrogen backbone (e.g., $CH_3-CH_2-CH_2-CH_3$) are referred to as **organic**. There are many kinds of **organic anions** in the body (e.g., $CH_3-CH_2-CH_2-COO^-$; note the negative charge). Sodium and potassium, as well as calcium, magnesium, and a few other substances, exist in nature as either ions (Na^+, K^+, Ca^{2+}, Mg^{2+}) or as uncharged atoms, but in the body they are found almost exclusively as ions. Therefore, when I say "sodium," "potassium," "calcium," and the like, I'm referring to the ions. Ions, or substances that release ions when they dissolve (like NaCl, which breaks apart into Na^+ and Cl^-), are sometimes called **electrolytes**.

---

[*]**Terminology.** In case you're wondering why the symbols Na and K are used, these come from the Latin names: Sodium = Natrium, Potassium = Kalium.

[**]**Mnemonic.** If you tend to mix up anion and cation, think of the "t" in cation as a stretched-out + sign, and the second letter of anion as standing for *negative*.

- Molecule: two or more atoms bound together by chemical bonds.
- Ion: an atom or molecule that carries an electrical charge.
- Cation: a positively charged (+) ion. Anion: a negatively charged (–) ion.
- Organic: having a carbon-hydrogen backbone (e.g., $-CH_2-CH_2-CH_2-$).
- Know these: Sodium (Na^+), Chloride (Cl^-), Potassium (K^+), Bicarbonate (HCO_3^-), Carbon dioxide (CO_2).
- Electrolyte: another name for ion, or for a substance that releases ions when dissolved (e.g., $NaCl \longrightarrow Na^+ + Cl^-$).

Body Fluids

In the body, all water is in the form of aqueous (water-based) solutions, which are referred to generically as **body fluids**. A large number of molecules and ions are dissolved in these solutions. The body fluids exist in two main locations: inside cells and outside cells. Fluid inside cells is called **intracellular fluid (ICF).** Fluid outside cells is called **extracellular fluid (ECF).** The extracellular fluid itself has two main components: **blood plasma** and **interstitial fluid.** Blood plasma is the fluid located inside blood vessels; it is the liquid medium in which blood cells and platelets are suspended. Interstitial fluid, which exists outside of the blood vessels, is located in the interstices (small spaces) between cells.

- ECF: Extracellular fluid. Fluid inside body but outside of cells.
- ECF = Blood plasma + interstitial fluid.
- ICF: Intracellular fluid. Fluid inside cells.

Concentrations

You can indicate the concentration of something by putting its chemical formula in brackets. For example, $[HCO_3^-]$ indicates bicarbonate concentration. Sometimes whole words are written in brackets. For example, [anion] indicates the total concentration of all anions in a solution, and [aldosterone] indicates the concentration of the hormone aldosterone. In the body fluids, the concentration of many molecules and ions is expressed in **millimoles per liter**, abbreviated as **mmol/l**. For example, if you write "$[K^+]$ = 4 mmol/l," you're indicating that the potassium concentration is 4 millimoles per liter. The term millimole refers to a specific, large number of particles, roughly 6×10^{20} (i.e., 6 followed by 20 zeros: 600,000,000,000,000,000,000). Therefore, a solution whose concentration is 1 mmol/l has about 6×10^{20} molecules or ions dissolved in one liter of fluid. You don't need to remember this number, but I want to give you a concrete sense of what the units refer to.

Some labs report concentrations of ions in **milli*equivalents* per liter**, abbreviated as **meq/l**, instead of mmol/l. A meq/l refers to a mmol/l *of electrical charges*. When an ion carries a single electrical charge, the concentration is the same whether stated in mmol/l or meq/l. For example, 1 mmol/l of Na^+ equals 1 meq/l because it has one mmol/l of charges. In contrast, 1 mmol/l of calcium ions (Ca^{2+}) equals

2 meq/l because each Ca^{2+} has two electrical charges. In this book, meq/l is used only in those few instances when it's necessary to refer to charges.

> • Concentration is indicated with brackets: $[K^+]$, $[Na^+]$, and $[HCO_3^-]$.
> • Concentration is often given in millimoles per liter, abbreviated as mmol/l.

Hydrogen Ions

The common hydrogen atom (atomic symbol H) has one proton, one electron, and no neutrons. If this atom loses its electron, a bare proton remains. This bare proton, which carries a single positive charge, is symbolized **H^+**. It can be called either a **hydrogen ion** or, simply, a **proton**. If you want to talk about the hydrogen ion concentration in a solution, you can simply write **$[H^+]$**. Solutions with a relatively high $[H^+]$ are said to be **acidic**. Solutions with a relatively low $[H^+]$ are said to be **basic** or **alkaline**. "Basic" and "alkaline" mean the same thing and can be used interchangeably.

> • H^+: Hydrogen ion (a.k.a. proton). Carries a positive charge.
> • $[H^+]$: Hydrogen ion concentration (a.k.a. proton concentration).
> • Acidic: Refers to a solution with a relatively high $[H^+]$.
> • Basic (or alkaline): Refers to a solution with a relatively low $[H^+]$.

Acid-Base

The term **"acid-base"** (as in "acid-base physiology" or "acid-base disturbance") refers to anything having to do with the regulation of $[H^+]$ in the body fluids.

The pH Scale

The pH scale provides a convenient way to talk about the $[H^+]$ of a solution. It is often used because actual $[H^+]$ values can involve long numbers. Using the pH scale lets you describe $[H^+]$ using just two or three digits. The pH scale has two important features. First, the scale is *inverse*. This means that a low pH indicates a high $[H^+]$, and a high pH indicates a low $[H^+]$. Therefore, a solution with a low pH is acidic, and a solution with a high pH is basic (or alkaline). Second, the pH scale is *logarithmic*, using 10 as its base. This means that a one-unit change in pH indicates a ten-fold change in $[H^+]$. Examples: If pH falls from 7 to 6, then $[H^+]$ has gone up ten times. If pH rises from 6 to 9, then $[H^+]$ has decreased 1000 times (10 x 10 x 10).*

---

*$*$**Terminology.** The term pH is actually a shorthand for $p[H^+]$, with the "p" indicating an inverse logarithmic relationship. Some writers italicize the p, like this: *p*H. The meaning is the same with or without italics.

The term pH can be defined mathematically in two ways. You don't need to remember these definitions for clinical purposes, but they're still worth understanding in a general way:

$$pH = \log (1/[H^+]) \qquad OR \qquad pH = -\log [H^+]$$

In the first definition, notice the $1/[H^+]$. This term indicates the inverse relationship. As $[H^+]$, the denominator, increases, the value of the fraction decreases—and pH decreases with it. So here you see the inverse nature of the pH scale built into the mathematical definition. In the second definition, the $1/[H^+]$ has been replaced by a simple $[H^+]$. However, the inverse relationship is maintained because a negative sign is placed before "log"—and a negative log is the same as the log of a reciprocal (one over something). That is, $-\log x = \log 1/x$. Therefore, the two definitions are mathematically identical. These two formulas tell you, mathematically, what you already know: that the pH scale is both inverse and logarithmic.

As I said, you don't need to remember these definitions, but one small fact is worth knowing: the log of 2 is nearly equal to 0.3. This seemingly obscure fact is important because it means that *if pH changes by 0.3, [H⁺] has changed by roughly a factor of two—either doubling or halving.* So, if pH rises from 7.4 to 7.7, $[H^+]$ is halved. If pH falls from 7.4 to 6.8, $[H^+]$ has increased four times. In this change from 7.4 to 6.8, notice that pH is reduced by 0.6, or 0.3 + 0.3. The first reduction of 0.3 means $[H^+]$ doubles. The second reduction of 0.3 means $[H^+]$ doubles again—in all, a four-fold change.

You've probably heard that the pH scale runs from 0 (most acidic) to 14 (most basic). You've probably also heard that pH 7 is neutral, that pH values below 7 are acidic, and that pH values above 7 are alkaline (or basic). These statements are reasonably accurate. As a practical matter, it's fine to think of them as true, though in reality they are slight simplifications.*

- Low pH = high [H+] = acidic.
- High pH = low [H+] = basic (alkaline).
- As pH decreases, [H+] increases.
- If pH changes by 1, [H+] has changed by a factor of 10.
- If pH changes by 0.3, [H+] has doubled or halved.

Why the [H⁺] (and pH) of Body Fluids Is Important

The body is highly sensitive to small changes in $[H^+]$ in its internal fluids. To understand why this is so takes some explanation. Because opposite charges attract, protons can bind to negatively charged (anionic) parts of large molecules such as proteins. (Many large molecules, especially proteins, have parts that carry an

---

*__Going further.__ It is theoretically possible for a solution to have a pH below 0 or above 14, though you're unlikely to encounter such extreme values even in a research laboratory. Neutral pH can actually deviate slightly from 7, depending on the temperature and chemical composition of the solution.

electrical charge.) The proton's small size makes it highly mobile and also gives it a high charge density (i.e., a high ratio of charge to volume), both of which increase the proton's ability to move to, and bind with, anionic regions of large molecules.

This kind of proton binding is reversible and depends on the pH of the solution. When the solution's [H⁺] rises (a fall in pH), there are more protons moving randomly and bumping into things, including the anionic sites. When a proton collides with an anionic site, it can bind to the site. The result is that the negative charge of the site is balanced by the proton's positive charge, giving the site a net charge of zero. Conversely, when [H⁺] falls (a rise in pH), there are fewer protons moving randomly and bumping into things. So fewer anionic sites are occupied by protons, and the sites thus retain their original negative charge. Thus, changes in body fluid pH can affect electrical charges on molecules throughout the body.

These alterations in the electrical charge on molecules can have major physiological effects. Proteins, such as enzymes, are especially vulnerable, because their three-dimensional structure is influenced by the charges on their constituent amino acids.* And alterations in a protein's three-dimensional structure can affect its function. For example, the shape and charge configuration of an enzyme must conform to the shape and charge configuration of the molecules the enzyme acts upon—like a glove fits on a hand. Therefore, when pH is abnormal, the fit is less precise and enzyme activity may be impaired. Likewise, the shape of structural proteins, which keep the cell's form and internal architecture intact, may be altered. The activity of protein channels and pumps, which carry ions and molecules across cell membranes, may also be altered. Changes in pH have other effects as well.**

The normal pH of arterial blood is 7.4. That is, normal blood plasma is mildly alkaline. The entire body system is tuned to function at this plasma pH, and marked alterations in pH are dangerous. In general, an arterial pH lower than approximately 6.8, or higher than approximately 7.8, is incompatible with human life and thus often lethal.

- Hydrogen ions (protons) can bind to molecules.
- Proton binding changes the charge on amino acids in proteins throughout the body, which can alter the structure and function of the proteins.
- Normal arterial pH is 7.4

---

*Reminder.** All proteins are made of amino acids that are strung together in a long chain. This chain twists and bunches up on itself in specific ways depending on electrical attractions, repulsions, and other forces.

** **Clinical note.** For example, when pH rises (a decrease in [H⁺]), additional anionic sites on plasma albumin molecules (which under normal conditions are bound to protons) are exposed to the body fluids. Some of these newly exposed negative sites attract and bind calcium ions (Ca²⁺) in the plasma, thus lowering the concentration of physiologically active "free" (unbound) calcium ions in the body fluids. The fall in [Ca²⁺] can cause a condition called tetany, which is characterized by peri-oral numbness, tingling of fingers and toes, and spasms of the flexor muscles of the wrists and ankles (carpopedal spasms). The fall in [Ca²⁺] can also decrease both vascular tone and cardiac contractility, both of which can contribute to a fall in blood pressure.

Electroneutrality

So far, I've used the word *neutral* to refer to the acid-base status of a solution. In that context, neutral, and the related word *neutrality*, mean the solution is neither acidic nor basic; the pH is intermediate. However, the word neutral can also be used in a different way: to refer to *electrical* neutrality. A solution that is electrically neutral, or *electroneutral*, is one in which the total number of positive and negative charges on dissolved ions is equal. The ECF (extracellular fluid) is an electroneutral solution, in that the sum of positive charges on Na^+, K^+, and the other dissolved cations equals the sum of negative charges on Cl^-, HCO_3^-, and the other dissolved anions. The ICF (intracellular fluid) is electroneutral, too. Actually, it turns out that *all* solutions are electrically neutral. ECF, ICF, saliva, sweat, and urine, as well as intravenous solutions, seawater, maple syrup, and even gasoline—all are electroneutral. The condition of electroneutrality is so inviolable that it is sometimes called the **Law of Electroneutrality**. This law holds true because it takes a tremendous amount of energy to separate positive and negative charges. For example, to prepare just 1/100 milliliter (1/5 of a typical drop) of a solution that has just 0.0001 mmol/l more positive than negative charges requires over a half million volts.

> • Law of Electroneutrality: All solutions have an equal number of positive and negative charges. They are electrically neutral.

Acid and Base

An **acid** is defined as a substance that can release protons. You can also say that an acid donates or gives up protons; the meaning is the same. **Hydrochloric acid (HCl)** is considered an acid because when it dissolves in water it **dissociates** (breaks apart), releasing protons, like this: $HCl \rightarrow H^+ + Cl^-$. Conversely, a **base** is defined as a substance that binds protons. You can also say that a base accepts or removes protons; again, the meaning is the same. The **hydroxide ion (OH⁻)** is considered a base because it can accept a proton, forming water: $OH^- + H^+ \rightarrow H_2O$. **Sodium hydroxide (NaOH)** is also considered a base because when it dissolves in water it dissociates into sodium ions (Na^+) and hydroxide ions (OH^-), like this: $NaOH \rightarrow Na^+ + OH^-$. As before, the hydroxide ion accepts a proton, forming water ($OH^- + H^+ \rightarrow H_2O$).

On occasion, another set of definitions for acid and base is used. According to this alternate terminology, an acid is defined as a substance that reduces pH when added to a solution, and a base is defined as a substance that increases pH when added to a solution. We can call this the "pH definition" of acids and bases. These alternate definitions are useful because there are a few situations where a substance can lower pH without directly releasing protons. The most important example is carbon dioxide gas (CO_2). CO_2 obviously has no protons to donate but when it dissolves in water it can cause water molecules (H_2O) to release some of their protons, thereby lowering pH. We'll study this reaction of CO_2 in the next chapter.

- Acid: a substance that donates (or releases) protons. Alternate definition: a substance that lowers pH.
- Base: a substance that accepts (or picks up) protons. Alternate definition: a substance that raises pH.

Strong Acids

It is common to distinguish between two categories of acid: strong and weak. **Strong acids** are acids that give up almost all of their protons when they dissolve. They dissociate almost completely, leaving virtually none of the acid in its original form. Hydrochloric acid (HCl) is a classic example. When it dissolves in water, almost 100 percent of the molecules dissociate into separate hydrogen and chloride ions (HCl $\rightarrow$ H$^+$ + Cl$^-$). **Sulfuric acid (H$_2$SO$_4$)** is another strong acid. It releases two protons (H$_2$SO$_4$ $\rightarrow$ 2H$^+$ + SO$_4^{2-}$), leaving a **sulfate anion (SO$_4^{2-}$)**. When present in sufficient quantity, strong acids can markedly lower the pH of a solution. There are also many **organic acids** (acids that have carbon-hydrogen backbones), and these, too, are relatively strong and dissociate almost completely in many circumstances, including in the ECF. When organic acids dissociate, organic anions are left (organic acid $\rightarrow$ H$^+$ + organic anion$^-$). The best-known example is **lactic acid**. Lactic acid forms the **lactate** anion when it dissociates. We'll see the chemical structures of lactic acid and lactate later in the book (p. 70).

Weak Acids

In contrast to strong acids, **weak acids** give up only some of their protons, dissociating only partly when dissolved in water. That is, only some of the acid molecules release their protons. Before considering actual examples of weak acids, let's learn some terms by referring to a made-up weak acid, which I'll call HX. It will be our demonstration model. HX consists of two parts, H$^+$ and X$^-$, that are stuck together—in much the same way that H$^+$ and Cl$^-$ are stuck together in hydrochloric acid (HCl). When HX dissolves in water, it can dissociate like this:

$$HX \rightarrow H^+ + X^-$$

However, unlike HCl, only some of the HX dissociates when it dissolves. The rest remains just as it was, as HX. Thus, after a weak acid dissolves, there are appreciable quantities of both the HX and X$^-$ forms in solution (as well as H$^+$). The dissociated form of the acid (X$^-$) is sometimes termed the **conjugate base**.* The weak acid (HX) and its conjugate base (X$^-$) are identical in every respect except that the conjugate base is missing a proton (H$^+$). Sometimes the non-dissociated form of the weak acid (HX) is referred to as a **conjugate acid**.

---

*__Terminology.__ The adjective *conjugate* means "joined together." It is related to *conjugal*, which refers to marriage. You can think of a weak acid as a kind of marriage (albeit a temporary one) between a base and a proton.

- Strong acid: An acid that dissociates completely when dissolved.
- Weak acid: An acid that dissociates only partly when dissolved.
- Weak acid: can be represented by the generic (made up) molecule HX.
- Conjugate base (X⁻): A weak acid (HX) without its proton.

Let's now look at actual weak acids found in the body. Two examples are the plasma protein **albumin** and the red blood cell protein **hemoglobin**. Both these proteins can function as weak acids because they contain significant quantities of an amino acid called histidine. Part of histidine's structure is a chemical ring, which looks like this:

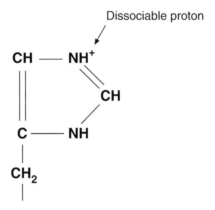

As you can see, this ring portion of histidine (chemically, called an imidazole ring) has a proton that can dissociate, like this:

Histidine's proton dissociates weakly, so the H^+ on only some histidine rings are released. In this figure, the structure on the left is the weak acid form (HX) and the structure on the right is the conjugate base form (X⁻). Imagine dozens of these ring structures sticking out from a protein chain, with each ring having its own weak-acid proton.*

---

* **Going further.** To give you a sense of how many acid groups can exist on a single protein molecule: of hemoglobin's 574 amino acids, 36 are histidine. In case you're wondering, the nitrogen atom (N) in the imidazole ring that releases the proton does not have a negative charge (as X⁻ does). However, it does have a "lone pair" of electrons: two electrons, not bound to any other atom, that are in the outermost region around the atom. These two electrons (not shown in the figure) give a partial negative charge to that area of the nitrogen atom, making it possible for the positively charged proton to attach weakly.

Describing an Acid's Strength: K and pK

It's useful to have a simple way to describe exactly how strong an acid is. One way to do this is with a value called the dissociation constant, symbolized **K**. The higher the K value, the stronger the acid. The lower the K, the weaker the acid. Because values of K can involve very long numbers, the letter "p" is applied to K—resulting in **pK**—in much the same way that "p" is used in the pH scale. Like pH, pK is an inverse measure. Therefore, strong acids have low pK values, and weak acids have high pK values. An acid whose pK is 3 is stronger than one whose pK is 4, and both of these acids are much stronger than one whose pK is 8. If two acids have the same pK, they are equal in strength and will dissociate to the same degree when dissolved in the same solution, even if they are different in other respects.

> - pK: A measure of an acid's strength, i.e., its tendency to release protons.
> - Lower pK = Stronger acid.
> - Higher pK = Weaker acid.

Buffers

A **buffer** is a chemical substance that helps stabilize the [H^+], and therefore the pH, of a solution. The word *buffer* comes from an archaic usage of the word *buff*, which means "to limit the shock of"—in this case, the shock of a pH change. Thus, a buffer is a pH shock absorber. A buffered solution is a solution that has a buffer dissolved in it. If you add a given quantity of a strong acid like HCl to a buffered solution, pH falls much less than it would if no buffer were present. If you add a given quantity of a strong base like NaOH to the solution, pH rises much less than it would if no buffer were present. *All body fluids, including blood plasma and urine, have buffers dissolved in them and thus are buffered solutions.* Note that buffers *minimize*, or *mitigate*, the change in pH that would otherwise occur, but they do not prevent the change entirely. So if you add strong acid to even a very well buffered solution, pH will still decrease somewhat.

A buffer is often referred to as a **buffer pair** because it consists of two main parts: a weak acid (HX) and its conjugate base (X^-). Let's see how this pair works together, using HX as our example. This time, I'll picture HX as being in equilibrium (indicated by the double arrow) with its conjugate base (X^-) and proton:

$$HX \rightleftharpoons X^- + H^+$$

By referring to this system as an equilibrium, I mean that the buffer is dissolved in water and that the concentrations of all the chemical species (HX, X^-, and H^+) are constant. (By chemical "species," I mean, simply, any chemical substance that participates in the equilibrium.) This constancy of concentrations makes sense since we're assuming that the weak acid has already dissociated as much as it's going to.

Let's see how this equilibrium (HX $\leftrightharpoons$ X$^-$ + H$^+$) functions as a buffer. Consider how the equilibrium responds when you add H$^+$ to the solution. For example, let's add a strong acid like HCl, which releases H$^+$ when it dissociates. As [H$^+$] starts to increase, some of the protons combine with dissolved X$^-$ via the reaction H$^+$ + X$^-$ $\rightarrow$ HX. This reaction occurs because an increase in [H$^+$] results in more random collisions between H$^+$ and X$^-$, and some of these collisions cause new HX molecules to form. Referring to the equilibrium (HX $\leftrightharpoons$ X$^-$ + H$^+$), we can say that the addition of protons shifts the equilibrium "to the left." This phrase means that that some of the chemical material on the right side of the double arrow (X$^-$ and H$^+$) is *converted into* the chemical substances on the *left* side of the double arrow (HX). After an equilibrium shifts left, more of the total mass in the system exists in the form on the left side of the arrows. Notice that this leftward shift takes some of the added free protons out of solution, thereby minimizing the rise in [H$^+$] that resulted from adding the HCl.

- Buffers: pH shock absorbers. Buffers minimize pH changes but don't prevent them entirely.
- Buffered solution: a solution with one or more buffers dissolved in it.
- If you add a strong acid or strong base to a buffered solution, pH changes less than it would have had no buffer been present.
- A buffer is sometimes called a buffer pair because it consists of two parts: a weak acid (HX) and its conjugate base (X$^-$).
- Buffers can be portrayed as an equilibrium: HX $\leftrightharpoons$ X$^-$ + H$^+$.
- If you add H$^+$ to a buffered solution, the equilibrium shifts left, removing some of the added H$^+$.

Le Chatelier's Principle

You can understand buffering even better if you're familiar with a chemical concept called **Le Chatelier's principle**. According to this principle, if you do something to change the concentration of any chemical species in an equilibrium (say, by deliberately adding or removing some of that species), the equilibrium *will automatically shift in a way that minimizes the change in concentration*. Put differently, the equilibrium system *resists* the change in concentration that you have tried to impose on it. To see how this works, let's again consider the buffer equilibrium:

$$HX \leftrightharpoons X^- + H^+$$

Let's again consider what happens if you add HCl to the solution, but this time, let's use Le Chatelier's principle to predict what will happen. When you add HCl, you are trying to impose a change in [H$^+$] on the solution (you are trying to increase [H^+]). Le Chatelier tells you that the equilibrium will resist that change. The equilibrium can do this only by shifting to the left, using up some of the added H^+ ions by combining them with X^-, forming HX.

Test your understanding by considering the reverse case: the addition of a strong base, like NaOH, to a buffered solution. *Pause here and use Le Chatelier's principle to figure out how the equilibrium reacts.* Once you have an answer, keep reading. Here you are attempting to impose a reduction in the [H^+] on the system. Le Chatelier tells you that the equilibrium will resist this change. It can do this only by generating additional H^+ to replace some of those removed by the NaOH. That is, the equilibrium must shift "to the right." This phrase means that some HX (on the left) is converted into additional X^- and H^+ (on the *right*). After an equilibrium shifts right, more of the total mass in the system exists in the forms on the right side of the double arrows. This shift to the right replaces some of the removed protons, thereby minimizing the fall in [H^+].

All these examples emphasize the fact that buffers minimize, or mitigate, pH changes, but don't entirely prevent them. Le Chatelier's principle gives you a shorthand way to predict how any buffer system will react when you add a strong acid or base.

Let's now revisit the ring portion of histidine, the weak acid structure in hemoglobin and albumin. Since the ring is a weak acid, it can function as a buffer. After histidine is dissolved in water, or in an aqueous solution like the ECF, the two forms of the ring exists in equilibrium, like this:

If [H^+] rises due to the addition of a strong acid like HCl, the equilibrium shifts left, towards the conjugate acid form (HX), thus removing some of the excess protons and helping to stabilize pH. Conversely, if [H^+] falls due to the addition of a strong base like NaOH, the equilibrium shifts right, towards the conjugate base form (X^-), thus replacing some of the lost protons, again stabilizing pH.

- Le Chatelier's principle: An equilibrium will shift in a way that minimizes any concentration change you try to impose on it. This principle helps you predict how buffers will function when you add a strong acid or base to a solution.

Effective Range of Buffers

Just as we can speak about the pK of an acid, we can speak about the pK of a buffer. This buffer pK is simply the pK of the weak acid in the buffer pair. For example, if a buffer has a pK of 5, you know that it consists of a weak acid whose pK is 5, along with the conjugate base of that weak acid. Buffers are most effective when their pKs are within about 1.5 units of the solution's pH. We can refer to this as the **1.5-unit rule**. For example, a buffer whose pK is 7 will be most effective in a solution whose pH is between 5.5 and 8.5 (1.5 units in either direction from the pK value). The 1.5-unit rule is relevant in the body. For example, this rule tells you that a buffer whose pK is 5 will be effective in acidic urine (which can have a pH as low as 4.4) but not in blood plasma (pH 7.4).

- 1.5-unit rule: A buffer works best when its pK value is within 1.5 units of the solution's pH.

Summary

Ions carry an electrical charge. Molecules are electrically neutral. Negatively charged ions can be called anions; positively charged ions can be called cations. Concentrations are indicated with brackets (e.g., $[Na^+]$ means sodium ion concentration) and are often expressed in millimoles per liter (mmol/l). The hydrogen ion, abbreviated H^+, can also be called a proton. Hydrogen ion concentration, also known as proton concentration, can be written as $[H^+]$. The pH is a measure of $[H^+]$. The pH scale is inverse, so a high pH means a low $[H^+]$, and a low pH means a high $[H^+]$. The pH scale is also base-10 logarithmic, meaning that a one-unit pH change indicates a 10-fold change in $[H^+]$. Thus, if pH changes from 6 to 8, you know that $[H^+]$ has decreased by a factor of 100. A pH change of 0.3 indicates a doubling or halving of $[H^+]$. The normal pH of arterial blood plasma is 7.4. The term acid-base refers to anything pertaining to the regulation of $[H^+]$ (and pH) of the body fluids. A strong acid is one that dissociates completely (or almost completely) when dissolved in solution. Examples of strong acids are hydrochloric acid (HCl) and sulfuric acid (H_2SO_4). A weak acid (sometimes symbolized HX) is an acid that dissociates only partly. This incomplete dissociation leaves appreciable quantities of both the original, undissociated acid form (HX), and the dissociated, or conjugate base, form (X^-) dissolved in solution. Examples of weak acids are the proteins albumin and hemoglobin. A buffer, which consists of a weak acid and its conjugate base in equilibrium, minimizes but does not entirely prevent changes in pH. Le Chatelier's principle describes how a buffer equilibrium automatically shifts in a way that resists any pH change you try to impose on a solution by adding a strong acid or base. You can describe the strength of acids using pK values: a low pK indicates a stronger acid, a high pK indicates a weaker acid. A buffer functions best when its pK value is within 1.5 units of the pH of the solution in which the buffer is dissolved ("the 1.5 unit rule").

Congratulations! This completes the review. You now have a great chemistry foundation for learning clinical acid-base. If you're confused about anything, spend a few more moments reviewing before you continue. And you can always refer back to this material if you need a quick reminder of something as you progress through the book. See you in Chapter 1!

The Chemical Foundation: The Bicarbonate Buffer System

In this first chapter, you'll learn about the most important buffer in the body: the bicarbonate buffer system. The rest of this book builds directly on the concepts presented here. The two main components of this buffer system are the bicarbonate ion (HCO_3^-), usually known simply as bicarbonate, and dissolved carbon dioxide gas (CO_2). Since HCO_3^- and CO_2 both play key roles, the buffer is sometimes called the bicarbonate–carbon dioxide buffer, but most people call it just the **bicarbonate buffer**. Because this buffer is so important, we'll study it very systematically. We'll start by seeing how CO_2 dissolves in water. Starting at that point lets us review the meaning of the term PCO_2, which is essential for understanding both the bicarbonate buffer and pulmonary function in general. At the end of the chapter, we'll briefly consider buffers other than the bicarbonate system.

How Carbon Dioxide Dissolves in Water

Atmospheric pressure at sea level is about 760 millimeters of mercury (abbreviated as mm Hg), meaning that the pressure exerted by the air can support a column of mercury 760 mm high. This pressure results from a vast number of randomly moving air molecules, which continually strike and thus push against the surface of objects. This pressure is experienced by any surface in contact with the air. Air is a mixture of gases (nitrogen, oxygen, carbon dioxide, etc.), meaning that the molecules of the various gases are completely intermingled with one another. In a mixture like this, each type of gas contributes part of the total pressure. The pressure contributed by a single type of gas in a gas mixture is called the **partial pressure**, since it is the *part* of the total pressure exerted by that one type of gas. To find the partial pressure of a gas, multiply the total pressure of the gas mixture by the fraction of the mixture accounted for by the gas in question. For example, if we create a gas mixture in which 10 percent of the molecules are carbon dioxide (CO_2), and the total pressure of the mixture is 1 atmosphere (760 mm Hg), the partial pressure of CO_2 is 0.10 x 760 = 76. Partial pressure is symbolized **P**, so in this example you can say that PCO_2 is 76 mm Hg or, simply, 76, with the units left unstated.*

---

* **Terminology.** To designate partial pressure, some writers use a small p (pCO_2) or put the P in italics (either PCO_2 or pCO_2). Other writers use a capital P but put the chemical formula of the gas in subscript (P_{CO_2}). All these abbreviations mean the same thing.

Let's now see what happens when a liquid, for example, water or an aqueous (water-based) solution, comes in contact with a gas. Scan the following figure, then keep reading.

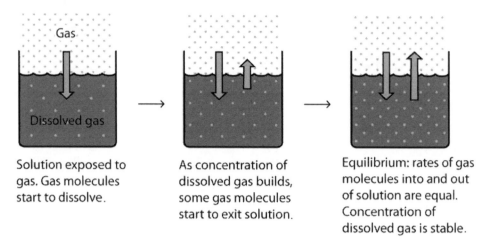

Solution exposed to gas. Gas molecules start to dissolve.

As concentration of dissolved gas builds, some gas molecules start to exit solution.

Equilibrium: rates of gas molecules into and out of solution are equal. Concentration of dissolved gas is stable.

The beaker on the left shows what happens when the liquid is first exposed to the gas. Notice that some of the randomly moving gas molecules strike the liquid's surface, penetrate the surface, and dissolve into the liquid. As the concentration of the dissolved gas molecules increases (middle beaker), some of the dissolved gas molecules, due to their own random movements, start to exit the solution. Eventually, as more and more gas molecules dissolve into the solution, the concentration of dissolved gas increases to the point where the rate of gas molecules exiting the solution equals the rate of gas molecules entering the solution (right beaker). At that point, the concentration of dissolved gas becomes stable and constant. In a mixture of gases, this kind of equilibrium is reached for each gas in the mixture.

Now, imagine that, after equilibrium is reached for a particular gas in the gas mixture, you increase the partial pressure of that gas (so that more of those gas molecules are bouncing around and striking the surface of the liquid). What happens? More of those molecules dissolve, and the concentration of that dissolved gas in the solution rises to a new, higher equilibrium level. Conversely, if you lower the partial pressure of the gas, the concentration of the dissolved gas decreases to a new equilibrium level. So, a higher partial pressure results in a higher concentration of the dissolved gas. We thus have a general rule: the concentration of a dissolved gas in a solution is *proportional* to the partial pressure of the gas in contact with the solution. You can refer to the concentration of dissolved gas using brackets, just as you would for the concentration of other molecules or ions dissolved in a solution. For example, you can indicate the concentration of dissolved CO_2 gas as $[CO_2]$. Therefore, you can say that if the partial pressure of carbon dioxide (PCO_2) in a gas mixture increases, then $[CO_2]$ in the solution increases. If the PCO_2 of a gas mixture decreases, then $[CO_2]$ in the solution decreases.* This figure summarizes the main point:

---

* **Hint.** The CO_2 in solution is fully dissolved, meaning the CO_2 molecules are well dispersed among the water molecules. The water remains perfectly clear. There are no bubbles.

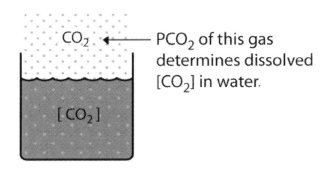

PCO_2 of this gas determines dissolved $[CO_2]$ in water.

So far, you know that the concentration of a dissolved gas will rise or fall in response to changes in the partial pressure of the gas in contact with the solution. But you still don't know the actual concentration of the dissolved gas. To find this concentration, you need to know the **solubility constant**. This constant tells you how much gas dissolves for each 1 mm Hg of partial pressure of that gas. For CO_2 in an aqueous solution like extracellular fluid (ECF) at body temperature, the constant is:

$$0.03 \text{ mmol}/\text{l}/\text{mm Hg}$$

This constant tells you that for each 1 mm Hg partial pressure of CO_2 in the air, dissolved $[CO_2]$ will be 0.03 millimoles per liter. You can also write this constant as 0.03 mmol/l *per* mm Hg. This form makes it a bit clearer that you get a concentration of 0.03 mmol/l *for each* 1 mm Hg of partial pressure. Using this constant, you can see:

If PCO_2 is 10 mm Hg, $[CO_2]$ will be 10 x 0.03 = 0.3 mmol/l
If PCO_2 is 100 mm Hg, $[CO_2]$ will be 100 x 0.03 = 3 mmol/l
If PCO_2 is 40 mm Hg, $[CO_2]$ will be 40 x 0.03 = 1.2 mmol/l

Until now, I've used the term partial pressure to describe the pressure exerted by a gas on a surface, including the surface of a liquid. But the term partial pressure can also be used—as a kind of short hand—to talk about the *concentration* of a gas that is dissolved in a solution. To use the term in this way, you simply state the partial pressure *that would have been required* to produce the concentration in question. Thus, if a gas whose PCO_2 is 40 mm Hg reaches equilibrium with water in a beaker, you can say that the PCO_2 of the water is, likewise, 40 mm Hg. This is a shorthand way of saying that $[CO_2]$ is 1.2 mmol/l (40 x 0.03). This figure summarizes these points:

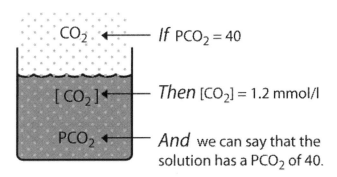

If $PCO_2 = 40$

Then $[CO_2] = 1.2$ mmol/l

And we can say that the solution has a PCO_2 of 40.

It is important to realize that a liquid can have many different gases dissolved in it at the same time (e.g., oxygen, carbon dioxide, nitrogen), just as it can have many non-gaseous substances dissolved in it at the same time (e.g., Na^+, K^+, glucose). Furthermore, each dissolved gas can have a different partial pressure. For example, arterial blood plasma typically has a PCO_2 of 40 and a PO_2 of 100. But for our purposes here, only CO_2 is important. As we'll soon see, the PCO_2 of normal arterial blood plasma (**arterial PCO_2**) is 40 mm Hg, which means that dissolved $[CO_2]$ is 1.2 mmol/l (because 40 x 0.03 = 1.2). If lung disease causes arterial PCO_2 to rise to 80 mm Hg, dissolved $[CO_2]$ in the blood plasma is twice the normal value, or 2.4 mmol/l. If hyperventilation causes arterial PCO_2 to fall to 20 mm Hg, dissolved $[CO_2]$ in the blood plasma is half of normal, or 0.6 mmol/l.

How Dissolved Carbon Dioxide Reacts with Water

When CO_2 first dissolves in water, its molecular structure is unchanged, even though it is now surrounded by water molecules (H_2O). However, the close proximity of the dissolved CO_2 to the water molecules makes it possible for some of the CO_2 to react chemically with H_2O, like this:

$$CO_2 + H_2O \rightarrow H_2CO_3$$

The product of this reaction, H_2CO_3, is called **carbonic acid**. It can give up a proton, like this:

$$H_2CO_3 \rightarrow H^+ + HCO_3^-$$

HCO_3^- is called the bicarbonate ion or, simply, **bicarbonate**. When we combine the above two reactions, we get:

$$CO_2 + H_2O \rightarrow H_2CO_3 \rightarrow H^+ + HCO_3^-$$

This two-step reaction shows that when CO_2 dissolves in water, CO_2 molecules can react chemically with water molecules, forming bicarbonate and protons, with carbonic acid acting as an intermediary. But it is important to realize that only a small fraction of the dissolved CO_2 molecules reacts in this way. The rest remains just as it was, as dissolved CO_2, surrounded by water but not reacting with it.

The reaction just shown can take several minutes to occur. (The formation of H_2CO_3, represented by the first arrow, is the slow step in the process.) However, the rate of the overall reaction can be greatly increased by an enzyme called **carbonic anhydrase**. Carbonic anhydrase speeds up the reaction by changing the reaction pathway (the route by which reactants get changed to products) to a faster one. The new pathway looks like this:

$$H_2O \rightarrow H^+ + OH^-$$
$$\downarrow$$
$$CO_2 \rightarrow HCO_3^-$$

In writing the reaction this way, I mean to indicate that, in the reaction catalyzed by carbonic anhydrase, carbonic acid is never produced at all. Instead, water is split, producing a proton and a hydroxide ion (OH^-). This hydroxide ion combines directly with the CO_2, producing HCO_3^-. These details are not essential to remember. The important point is that the reactants (CO_2, H_2O) and products (HCO_3^-, H^+) are the same whether or not carbonic acid is produced. Therefore, you can represent both the catalyzed (when carbonic anhydrase is present) and uncatalyzed (when carbonic anhydrase is not present) reactions with a single summary reaction:

$$CO_2 + H_2O \rightarrow H^+ + HCO_3^-$$

Based on this summary reaction, we can say that carbon dioxide acts as an acid, since it leads to the release of a proton and thus lowers the pH of the solution.* Since only a fraction of the dissolved carbon dioxide reacts with water (most remains simply as dissolved CO_2) we can think of CO_2 as a *weak* acid. The pK of CO_2, acting as an acid, is 6.1.

How Dissolved Carbon Dioxide and Bicarbonate Act as a Buffer

Let's now write the above summary reaction as an equilibrium:

$$CO_2 + H_2O \leftrightharpoons H^+ + HCO_3^-$$

Looking at this equilibrium, we can say that bicarbonate acts as the conjugate base of the weak acid CO_2. We thus have a buffer system: a weak acid and its conjugate base. We can call this system the bicarbonate-carbon dioxide buffer, though it is usually called simply the bicarbonate buffer. This buffer does not precisely fit the standard buffer pattern ($HX \leftrightharpoons X^- + H^+$) but it reacts to pH changes like any other buffer. When H^+ ions are added to the solution from strong acids, the equilibrium shifts to the left, meaning that some of the protons combine with HCO_3^-, forming CO_2 and H_2O, thereby minimizing the rise in $[H^+]$. Conversely, when H^+ are removed from the solution through the addition of a strong base, the equilibrium shifts right, meaning that some of the CO_2 and H_2O combine, releasing H^+ and thereby minimizing the fall in $[H^+]$. These shifts conform to Le Chatelier's principle.** They help stabilize $[H^+]$ and pH any time a strong acid or base is added.

*** Terminology.** The most common definition for an acid is a substance that releases a proton when it dissolves. But we can also define an acid as a substance that lowers pH when it dissolves, even if that substance does not itself release the proton (p. 6). CO_2 is an acid by this second definition.

**** Reminder.** Le Chatelier's principle tells you that a chemical equilibrium will shift in a way that minimizes a change in concentration that you try to impose on it (pp. 10–11). In this case, you've tried to change the $[H^+]$, and the equilibrium shifts in a way that limits the extent of that change.

Although the bicarbonate buffer is an equilibrium system, which is formally shown with a double arrow, it's sometimes easier to portray buffering reactions with a single arrow, that is, as simple reactions. For example, if HCl is added to the solution, and [H$^+$] rises, we can show the buffering of excess protons like this: $H^+ + HCO_3^- \rightarrow CO_2 + H_2O$. Conversely, if we add the strong base NaOH, and [H$^+$] falls, we can show the release of additional protons by the buffer like this: $CO_2 + H_2O \rightarrow H^+ + HCO_3^-$. Whether we show these buffering processes as a simple reaction (single arrow) or as equilibrium shifts (double arrow), the chemical events are the same.

Manipulating the Bicarbonate Buffer System to Regulate [H+]

Look again at the bicarbonate buffer equilibrium:

$$CO_2 + H_2O \leftrightharpoons H^+ + HCO_3^-$$

Let's see what happens to this equilibrium if, instead of changing [H$^+$], we change either PCO_2 or [HCO$_3^-$]. To predict the result, think of Le Chatelier's principle. First, visualize what happens if you dissolve additional CO_2 in the solution, thus raising the solution's PCO_2 (i.e., its [CO$_2$]). Consistent with Le Chatelier, which resists this rise in [CO$_2$], the equilibrium shifts to the right, lowering [CO$_2$] towards its starting level by converting some of the additional CO_2 into $H^+ + HCO_3^-$. As part of this equilibrium shift, [H$^+$] rises and pH falls because additional H$^+$ have been produced. Now consider what happens if you lower PCO_2. The equilibrium shifts left. This shift, again consistent with Le Chatelier, tends to increase [CO$_2$] towards its starting level by converting some H$^+$ and HCO$_3^-$ into CO_2 and H_2O. In the process, [H$^+$] falls and pH rises. As you can see, changing PCO_2 alters pH. Similar processes are at work when you change [HCO$_3^-$]. Increasing [HCO$_3^-$] shifts the equilibrium left and lowers [H$^+$], increasing pH. Decreasing [HCO$_3^-$] shifts the equilibrium right and increases [H$^+$], decreasing pH.*

Based on the ideas in the preceding paragraph, we can say the following:

> If you want to change the pH of a solution indirectly—without directly adding or removing protons—you can do so by changing either PCO_2 or [HCO$_3^-$].

This statement is crucially important because it is through this indirect approach that the body regulates pH. Specifically, the lung regulates the PCO_2 of the body fluids, and the kidney regulates the [HCO$_3^-$] of the body fluids. Thus, *it is through the regulation of PCO_2 (by the lung) and [HCO$_3^-$] (by the kidney) that the body sets the pH of blood and the rest of the ECF.* We'll study these pulmonary and renal processes in Chapters 2–4. Under normal conditions, the body maintains plasma

---

*__Hint.__ You can predict the same effects on pH by recognizing that CO_2 is an acid and HCO$_3^-$ is a base. Adding more acid (CO_2) acidifies (raises [H$^+$], lowers pH), whereas removing acid alkalinizes (lowers [H$^+$], raises pH). Adding more base (HCO$_3^-$) alkalinizes (lowers [H$^+$], raises pH), whereas removing base acidifies (raises [H$^+$], lowers pH).

[HCO$_3^-$] at about 24 mmol/l. As mentioned before, arterial PCO$_2$ is maintained at about 40 mm Hg (a [CO$_2$] of 1.2 mmol/l). At this [HCO$_3^-$] and PCO$_2$, pH is fixed at 7.4—the normal pH of arterial blood. If [HCO$_3^-$] or PCO$_2$ deviate from their normal levels, pH deviates as well.

A Final Word: Other Buffers in the Body

In addition to the bicarbonate buffer system, there are many less important buffers in the body, the so-called **non-bicarbonate buffers**. These include hemoglobin, albumin, and other protein molecules both inside and outside of cells. These proteins function as buffers because they are rich in the amino acid histidine, which as part of its structure has a chemical ring (imidazole) that possesses a weakly dissociable proton (p. 8). Another non-bicarbonate buffer is phosphate, which exists both free in the ECF and in the form of phosphate groups that are built into the structure of larger molecules (so-called "organic phosphates"). There are also buffers built into bones, which can come into play during chronic acidosis (a term I'll define fully in the next chapter).

Summary

In the bicarbonate buffer system, dissolved carbon dioxide gas (CO$_2$) acts as the weak acid, and bicarbonate (HCO$_3^-$) acts as the conjugate base. The overall buffer equilibrium is CO$_2$ + H$_2$O $\leftrightharpoons$ H$^+$ + HCO$_3^-$, which is the same whether or not the reaction is catalyzed by the enzyme carbonic anhydrase. This buffer equilibrium can function in two ways. First, if we change [H$^+$] by adding strong acid or strong base, the buffer equilibrium will shift to minimize the change in [H$^+$]. This is the traditional buffer function of minimizing changes in [H$^+$]. Second, if we change either [HCO$_3^-$] or PCO$_2$, the equilibrium will shift in a way that changes [H$^+$]. This second buffer function, which provides an indirect way to change and control pH, is of central importance in the body's pH regulation: by controlling [HCO$_3^-$] and PCO$_2$, the body regulates pH. Normal arterial [HCO$_3^-$] is about 24 mmol/l. Normal arterial dissolved [CO$_2$] is about 1.2 mmol/l, which can also be expressed as a PCO$_2$ of 40 mm Hg. At these normal levels of PCO$_2$ and [HCO$_3^-$], arterial pH is set at its normal level, 7.4. As we'll see in detail in Chapters 2–4, the kidney regulates [HCO$_3^-$] and the lung regulates PCO$_2$, thus making the kidney and lung the main organs of acid-base regulation.

Chapter 2

Overview of Acid-Base: A Balancing Act

In this chapter, we'll study the big picture of both normal and abnormal acid-base balance. By the time you finish the chapter, you'll be able to think clearly about acid-base balance in both healthy individuals and patients with serious acid-base disturbances. And you'll possess the vocabulary to communicate your insights to others. You'll also have an excellent framework for integrating the details of acid-base that you'll encounter in subsequent chapters.

Normal Acid-Base: The Body's Overall Acid-Base System

The three variables most relevant to acid-base balance are pH, bicarbonate concentration ($[HCO_3^-]$), and PCO_2. These are sometimes called the three acid-base variables. The normal pH of arterial blood plasma is **7.40**, which is often stated simply as **7.4**. The normal range is **7.35–7.45**, with slight variations among hospital laboratories. The 7.40 value is the mid-point of the normal range and is sometimes thought of as the "classic" normal value. Within the 7.35–7.45 range, each person has his or her own specific set-point pH, or at least a narrow personal range. The normal $[HCO_3^-]$ of arterial plasma is **24 mmol/l**, with a normal range of about **21–27 mmol/l**. The normal PCO_2 of arterial plasma is **40 mm Hg**, with a normal range of about **35–45 mm Hg**.* The following table summarizes these normal arterial values.

Acid-Base Variables: Normal Values in Arterial Blood Plasma			
Variable	"Classic" normal value (mid-point of normal range)	Normal range (can vary slightly depending on the lab)	Units
pH	7.4	7.35–7.45	pH has no units.
$[HCO_3^-]$	24	21–27	mmol/l (or meq/l)
PCO_2	40	35–45	mm Hg

***Reminder.** Although the "P" in PCO_2 technically refers to the *pressure* exerted by a gas, you can use the term PCO_2 to speak about the *concentration* of dissolved CO_2 in a liquid (p. 17). That is how the term is commonly used in the clinical setting. If for any reason you want to convert PCO_2 into a mmol/l value for dissolved CO_2, just multiply PCO_2 by 0.03. For example, if PCO_2 is normal (40 mm Hg), multiply 40 x 0.03, which gives you 1.2 mmol/l. So 1.2 is the mmol/l equivalent of 40 mm Hg.

In Chapter 1, we saw that you can change the $[H^+]$, and hence the pH, of a solution by altering its PCO_2 or its $[HCO_3^-]$. You can understand this effect by looking at the bicarbonate buffer system: $CO_2 + H_2O \leftrightharpoons H^+ + HCO_3^-$. For instance, increasing $[HCO_3^-]$ pushes the equilibrium to the left, reducing $[H^+]$ (increasing pH). In contrast, increasing PCO_2 pushes the equilibrium to the right, increasing $[H^+]$ (reducing pH). You can visualize these effects on pH using the analogy of a balance. Take a moment to scan the following figure, and then keep reading:

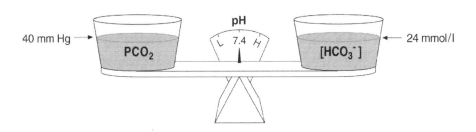

This is a simple but very useful illustration. Observe that the whole figure is set up so that you change pH by changing PCO_2 or $[HCO_3^-]$. You do not directly grab the pH needle and shift it right or left. Likewise, to keep pH stable, you don't grab the needle and hold it in place. Rather, you keep PCO_2 and $[HCO_3^-]$ constant, and pH remains stable as a consequence. Also observe that when PCO_2 is 40 and $[HCO_3^-]$ is 24, pH is 7.4—all the normal values.

To see how this figure works in practice, visualize what happens to the balance, and to pH, if you increase PCO_2. Notice that when PCO_2 increases, the level in the bucket rises, so the PCO_2 bucket gets heavier. That tips the scale to the left, lowering pH. Next, visualize what happens if you decrease PCO_2. When PCO_2 decreases, the level in the bucket falls, so the bucket weighs less. Therefore, the scale tips to the right, raising pH. For practice, visualize what happens if $[HCO_3^-]$ increases. Then visualize what happens if $[HCO_3^-]$ decreases. Confirm your answers here.*

This figure is important because the body's pH is regulated just as it is in the balance: through the maintenance of a normal PCO_2 by the lung and a normal $[HCO_3^-]$ by the kidney. *Thus, this figure portrays the body's overall system of pH regulation.* By adding a few pieces of information to the figure, we can summarize the main points covered so far in this chapter. Take a moment to absorb this figure:

---

*__Answer.__ If $[HCO_3^-]$ increases, the level in the bucket rises, so the $[HCO_3^-]$ bucket gets heavier. The scale tips to the right, increasing pH. If $[HCO_3^-]$ decreases, the level in the bucket goes down, so the bucket gets lighter. The scale tips left, decreasing pH.

How the Body Regulates Arterial pH

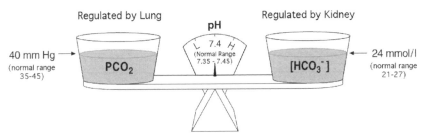

Body holds pH normal by keeping PCO_2 and $[HCO_3^-]$ stable.

The balance figure also serves another useful function: it portrays, in simple visual terms, the main message of a mathematical construct called the **Henderson-Hasselbalch ("H-H") equation**. The H-H equation looks like this:

pH = pK + log ([conjugate base]/[weak acid])

For clinical purposes, you don't need to know this equation in detail. But it's still worth spending a moment getting a sense of how the equation can apply to the bicarbonate buffer system. All buffers have two key chemical parts: a weak acid and its conjugate base. Notice that these parts form the denominator and numerator, respectively, in the final term of the H-H equation. In Chapter 1, we saw that, in the bicarbonate buffer system, dissolved CO_2 acts as the weak acid (that is, it acts to lower pH) and HCO_3^- acts as the conjugate base (that is, it acts to raise pH). You can see this by looking at balance illustration or, for that matter, the buffer equilibrium formula. What about pK? Recall that pK is a measure of acidic strength, the proton-releasing ability of an acid (p. 9). We saw in Chapter 1 that the pK of dissolved CO_2 is 6.1 (p. 19). Therefore, the H-H equation for the bicarbonate buffer system can be written like this:

$$pH = 6.1 + \log ([HCO_3^-]/[CO_2])$$

The normal values for $[HCO_3^-]$ and $[CO_2]$, measured in mmol/l, are about 24 and 1.2, respectively. If you plug these values into the equation, you get:

$$pH = 6.1 + \log (24/1.2)$$

If you realize that $24/1.2 = 20$, and you have a calculator handy (or happen to know that the log of $20 = 1.3*$), you can solve the equation like this:

$$pH = 6.1 + \log (24/1.2)$$
$$pH = 6.1 + \log 20$$
$$pH = 6.1 + 1.3$$
$$pH = 7.4$$

---

* **Math.** Mentally break 20 down into 10 x 2. When you work with logs, you multiply numbers by adding their logs. The log of 10 = 1. The log of 2 = 0.3. 20 = 1 + 0.3 = 1.3.

So, once again—this time mathematically—you see that when bicarbonate and dissolved CO_2 levels are normal, arterial pH is 7.4. If you change either $[HCO_3^-]$ or $[CO_2]$, the H-H equation lets you calculate the new pH.*

Let's now see how the balance figure fits in with the body's overall physiology. If the body were a simple container, like a glass beaker, regulating pH would be easy. You would adjust PCO_2 and $[HCO_3^-]$ and seal off the opening. PCO_2 and $[HCO_3^-]$ would stay constant and pH would never change. However, the body is not a simple container. Normal physiological processes continually act to alter the $[HCO_3^-]$ and PCO_2, and thus the pH, of the body fluids. For example, when you eat protein in the diet, sulfur atoms from the two sulfur-containing amino acids (cysteine and methionine) are metabolized to sulfuric acid (H_2SO_4). This acid dissociates into sulfate (SO_4^{2-}) and two protons ($H_2SO_4 \rightarrow SO_4^{2-} + 2H^+$). These protons combine with bicarbonate via the buffering reaction $H^+ + HCO_3^- \rightarrow CO_2 + H_2O$. This reaction consumes (i.e., uses up) bicarbonate and releases a small amount of CO_2.

If that were the end of the story, plasma $[HCO_3^-]$ would decrease, PCO_2 would increase, and—consistent with the balance figure—pH would fall. However, in reality, $[HCO_3^-]$ and PCO_2 change by only a trivial amount and only temporarily, and their values usually stay well within their normal ranges. The reason is that the kidneys replace the lost bicarbonate and the lungs eliminate the newly produced CO_2 (along with the much greater quantity of CO_2 produced at the tissues by aerobic metabolism). Thus, the regulation of pH is a dynamic balancing act between processes that alter $[HCO_3^-]$ and PCO_2, and processes—carried out by the kidney and lung—that return $[HCO_3^-]$ and PCO_2 to normal. It is only when this balancing act goes awry that $[HCO_3^-]$ or PCO_2, and hence pH, deviate markedly from their normal values.

For emphasis, I'll restate some key points in the following box:

> - The kidney and the lung are the two main organs of acid-base regulation.
> - The lung regulates PCO_2 and the kidney regulates $[HCO_3^-]$.
> - By modulating pulmonary (lung) and renal (kidney) activity, the body keeps arterial pH at its normal value.

Abnormal Acid-Base:
Speaking the Language of Clinical Acid-Base Disorders

When the body's pH regulation goes awry, regardless of the reason, the situation is called either an **acid-base disturbance** or an **acid-base disorder**. These terms are synonyms and can be used interchangeably. To discuss acid-base disturbances, you need to know four pairs of terms:

---

* **Hint.** If you still find the H-H equation confusing, don't worry. For most purposes, the balance illustration is all you need to know.

Acidemia & Alkalemia
Acidosis & Alkalosis
Respiratory & Metabolic
Simple & Mixed

Acidemia and Alkalemia

As I have mentioned before, the normal pH range for arterial blood plasma is 7.35–7.45. Anything outside of this range is abnormal. A pH below 7.35 is termed **acidemia**. A pH above 7.45 is termed **alkalemia**. The word root "-emia" means blood, as in anemia and ischemia. So, acidemia literally means "acid blood" and alkalemia means "alkaline blood." Notice that the terms acidemia and alkalemia don't tell you anything about the *cause* of the pH change. To talk about the cause of a pH change, the terms acidosis and alkalosis are used, as we'll now see.

Acidosis and Alkalosis

The word root "-osis" means pathologic condition or process, as in thrombosis and psychosis. **Acidosis** is a "pathologic acid process." It is a process that releases protons and lowers pH. Thus, an acidosis is what causes acidemia. **Alkalosis** is a "pathologic alkaline process." It removes protons and raises pH. Thus, an alkalosis is what causes alkalemia. There is no way to develop an acidemia except from an acidosis, and no way to develop an alkalemia except from an alkalosis. Clinically, if you detect an acidemia or alkalemia, you know that an acidosis or alkalosis is present: "-emia" implies "-osis." If a pH measurement tells you that acidemia is present, you know that an acidosis exists. If a pH measurement tells you that alkalemia is present, you know that an alkalosis is present.

Respiratory and Metabolic

To understand the terms respiratory and metabolic, it's useful to look again at the balance figure:

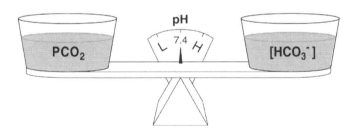

Notice that alterations in pH can be understood as arising from a change in either PCO_2 or $[HCO_3^-]$. This makes it useful to distinguish between two main groups of acid-base disorders: those caused by PCO_2 changes and those caused by $[HCO_3^-]$ changes. Respiratory and metabolic are labels used to distinguish between these two main groups. **Respiratory** is used to indicate an acidosis or alkalosis that involves a pathologic change in PCO_2. **Metabolic** is used to indicate an acidosis or alkalosis that involves a pathologic change in $[HCO_3^-]$. Therefore, when you see "respiratory," think PCO_2. And when you see "metabolic," think $[HCO_3^-]$.*

All acidoses and alkaloses are either respiratory or metabolic. Thus, there are four main types of acid-base disturbances:

Respiratory acidosis is a pathologic process that increases PCO_2 (↑ **PCO₂**)
Respiratory alkalosis is a pathologic process that decreases PCO_2 (↓ **PCO₂**)
Metabolic acidosis is a pathologic process that decreases $[HCO_3^-]$ (↓ **[HCO₃⁻]**)
Metabolic alkalosis is a pathologic process that increases $[HCO_3^-]$ (↑ **[HCO₃⁻]**)

These four abnormal conditions are called the **primary acid-base disturbances**. All acid-base disturbances, no matter what the underlying causes, fall under the heading of one of these four primary disturbances. I'll use balance figures to reinforce these concepts visually. Spend a moment looking them over before continuing:

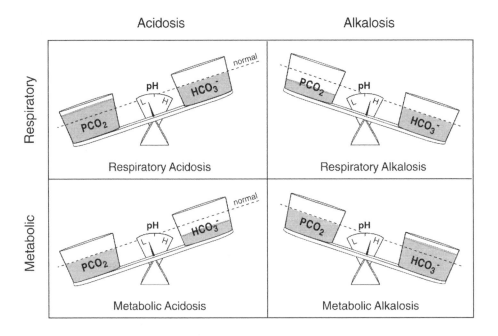

In Chapters 6–10 , we'll study specific disease states that cause each of the primary acid-base disturbances. Here I'll briefly mention a few diseases without explaining them, as a way to start you thinking clinically about the four primary disturbances:

---

* **Terminology.** As it is commonly used in biology, *metabolic* refers to the processes of metabolism (sometimes called "intermediary metabolism"), the biochemical pathways that build up, break down, or otherwise alter the structure of molecules in the body. This meaning of metabolism has no necessary connection to the term metabolic as it is used in acid-base. Thus, it's best to think of *metabolic* as having two distinct meanings, one of which pertains to metabolism and one of which pertains to acid-base disturbances.

- ▸ If chronic obstructive pulmonary disease (COPD) increases arterial PCO_2 to 55 mm Hg (from 40), a respiratory acidosis is present.
- ▸ If pain or anxiety causes a patient to hyperventilate, reducing arterial PCO_2 to 20, a respiratory alkalosis is present.
- ▸ If renal failure causes plasma $[HCO_3^-]$ to decrease to 16 mmol/l (from 24), metabolic acidosis is present.
- ▸ If diabetic ketoacidosis reduces $[HCO_3^-]$ to 12 mmol/l, metabolic acidosis is present.
- ▸ If severe vomiting increases plasma $[HCO_3^-]$ to 37 mmol/l, metabolic alkalosis is present.

Simple and Mixed

As we have just seen, there are four primary acid-base disturbances: metabolic acidosis, metabolic alkalosis, respiratory acidosis, and respiratory alkalosis. A patient who has *one* of the four primary disturbances is said to have a **simple disturbance**. If a patient has *more than one* primary disturbance at the same time, a **mixed** or **complex** disturbance (either term can be used) is said to be present. For example, if a patient has both respiratory acidosis (high PCO_2) and metabolic acidosis (low $[HCO_3^-]$), a mixed disturbance is present.*

Mixed disturbances usually involve *two* primary disorders (though three or even four are occasionally present). When both these disorders are acidoses or both are alkaloses—say, a respiratory *alkalosis* plus a metabolic *alkalosis*—the pH changes are additive. In this situation, the pH change can be severe and life threatening even if the component primary disorders are not by themselves severe. Conversely, when an *acidosis* and an *alkalosis* occur together, the effects on pH are opposite and therefore offset each other, so the actual pH change is usually modest even when the component disorders are severe. An example is a mixed metabolic acidosis and respiratory alkalosis. In this situation, the final pH can be either high or low, depending on which of the component disorders is most severe. Sometimes, the effects on pH exactly cancel, resulting in a normal pH.

As with pH, the final $[HCO_3^-]$ in a mixed disturbance can also reflect the additive or offsetting effects of the individual disturbances. For example, when a metabolic acidosis (low $[HCO_3^-]$) and metabolic alkalosis (high $[HCO_3^-]$) occur at the same time, the final $[HCO_3^-]$ can be low, high, or normal, depending on the relative severities of the two disturbances.

Later in this book, I'll say much more about mixed disturbances, and you'll gain experience working practice problems involving them.

---

* **Terminology.** Mixed disturbances can also take the form of two different causes of the same primary acid-base disturbance. Consider a patient with metabolic acidosis from chronic renal failure who then develops metabolic acidosis from uncontrolled type 1 diabetes (diabetic ketoacidosis). This patient has two different causes of metabolic acidosis and thus is considered to have a mixed disturbance.

Summary

In a healthy person, arterial PCO_2 is about 40 mm Hg (normal range 35–45) and arterial $[HCO_3^-]$ is about 24 mmol/l (normal range 21–27). When these levels are maintained, arterial plasma pH is normal, 7.4 (normal range 7.35–7.45). Changes in either PCO_2 or $[HCO_3^-]$ affect pH. The direction of these changes can be determined by considering the bicarbonate buffer equilibrium (CO_2 + $H_2O \leftrightharpoons H^+ + HCO_3^-$) or by looking at the balance figure (p. 24). Acidemia is defined as a low blood pH, and alkalemia is defined as a high blood pH. Acidosis and alkalosis are pathophysiologic processes that cause, respectively, acidemia and alkalemia. Respiratory and metabolic are adjectives used to modify the terms acidosis and alkalosis. Respiratory indicates a pathologic change in PCO_2, whereas metabolic indicates a pathologic change in plasma $[HCO_3^-]$. There are four primary acid-base disorders: metabolic acidosis (pathologic ↓ in $[HCO_3^-]$), metabolic alkalosis (pathologic ↑ in $[HCO_3^-]$), respiratory acidosis (pathologic ↑ in PCO_2), respiratory alkalosis (pathologic ↓ in PCO_2). A simple disturbance refers to the presence of one of these four primary disturbances. A mixed (a.k.a. complex) disturbance refers to the simultaneous presence of two or more primary disturbances.

Chapter 3

Acid-Base Physiology: The Lung

In this chapter, we'll study how, in healthy persons, the body keeps arterial PCO_2 (the concentration of dissolved CO_2 gas) stable at about 40 mm Hg. As you'll see, the respiratory system achieves this stable level by matching alveolar ventilation to carbon dioxide production. To set the stage, we'll study how the PCO_2 of blood changes as it circulates through the cardiovascular system. Understanding this chapter will give you a solid foundation for studying the respiratory acid-base disorders (i.e., respiratory acidosis and respiratory alkalosis).

PCO_2 and the Cardiovascular Circuit

Inside cells, food molecules, especially carbohydrates and fats, are broken down to produce ATP for energy, with carbon dioxide formed as a byproduct. Each day, about 15,000 millimoles of CO_2 are produced at the tissues and are carried in blood to the lung for elimination. Look over the following figure, and then refer back to it as you keep reading. Be sure to examine the key on the right, so you can see what PCO_2 is at various locations in the circulatory system. All these PCO_2 values are for a healthy person; PCO_2 will be higher throughout the circuit in respiratory acidosis and lower in respiratory alkalosis.

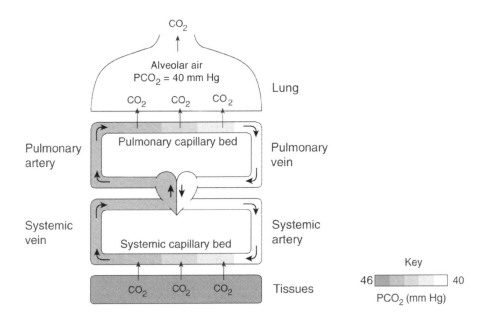

Let's start with blood leaving the lung in the pulmonary vein. Notice in the figure (and key) that this blood has a PCO_2 of 40 mm Hg. The PCO_2 stays at this level as the blood moves through the left side of the heart (right side of the figure), passes through systemic arteries, and is delivered to the tissues via the systemic capillaries. PCO_2 in the tissues, where the CO_2 is produced, is about 46 mm Hg. Since blood entering the capillaries has a PCO_2 of 40, there is diffusion gradient of about 6 mm Hg driving the entry of CO_2 into capillary blood. By the end of the tissue capillaries, blood PCO_2 has risen by 5 mm Hg to about 45. PCO_2 stays at this level as blood moves through the systemic veins, the right (pulmonary) side of the heart, and the pulmonary arteries.

At the lung, blood enters the pulmonary capillaries. Notice in the figure that air in the lung's alveoli ("alveolar air") has a PCO_2 of about 40. Because blood entering the pulmonary capillaries has a PCO_2 of 45, there is a 5 mm Hg diffusion gradient that drives the exit of CO_2 from pulmonary capillary blood into the lung's air spaces. Although CO_2 is constantly entering the lung's air spaces from the capillary blood, normal ventilation serves to eliminate this CO_2 into the atmosphere. This elimination keeps the PCO_2 of alveolar air constant at 40, thus allowing for on-going diffusion of CO_2 from blood into the air spaces. The exit of CO_2 from pulmonary capillary blood causes the blood's PCO_2 to fall from 45 to 40. The circuit starts again as blood exits the lung and enters the pulmonary veins.

We'll end this part of the chapter with a close-up view of a single alveolus and pulmonary capillary. Take a moment to study it before proceeding. Doing so will let you review much of what we just discussed, from a very different perspective. To give you a sense of the scale, an alveolus is about a quarter of a millimeter in diameter. Each of the two lungs has about 250 million alveoli.

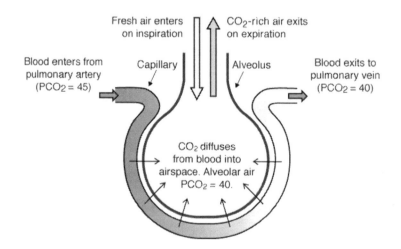

The Regulation of Arterial PCO_2

You don't need to know many respiratory definitions for this book, but it's useful to have a strong "gut sense" of what alveolar ventilation is and how it fits in with other measures of ventilation. A good way to develop this sense is to think through a few key terms. So take a moment to read this shaded box before continuing:

Some Terms Related to Ventilation

Total ventilation, also known as minute ventilation, is the broadest measure of ventilation (typical value = 7.5 liters/minute). These terms refer to air movement into and out of the respiratory tree as a whole. If you put your hand in front of your nose and mouth to feel your breath, total ventilation, a.k.a. minute ventilation, is what you're feeling. In this book, I generally say "total ventilation," but don't hesitate to mentally translate that to "minute ventilation" if you prefer.*

Alveolar ventilation (typical value = 5 liters/min) is the part of total ventilation that reaches the alveoli-rich distal respiratory tree, where gas exchange occurs. Air gets to the alveolar region via the conducting airways (think: ducts), including trachea, main bronchi, and many levels of bronchioles. The air space in these conducting airways (typically, about 150 ml in total) is referred to as dead space. In this context, "dead" means simply "not participating in gas exchange." It follows that dead space ventilation (typical value = 2.5 liters/min) is the part of total ventilation that moves in and out of conducting airways but does not reach the alveoli.

Let's see how this all fits together. Of the total amount of air entering the respiratory tree (total ventilation), part reaches the alveoli (alveolar ventilation) and part never gets beyond the conducting airways (dead space ventilation). Therefore:

Total ventilation = Alveolar ventilation + Dead space ventilation

If you plug in the typical values mentioned above (7.5, 5.0, 2.5), you'll see that the math works out. If you rearrange this equation, you can define alveolar ventilation, like this:

Alveolar ventilation = Total ventilation – Dead Space ventilation

This equation tells you that alveolar ventilation equals total ventilation minus that portion of total ventilation that remains in the conducting airways and therefore doesn't make it to the alveoli. This equation is actually pretty obvious once you understand what the three terms mean.

Alveolar ventilation usually changes roughly in parallel with total ventilation. That is, when total ventilation increases, alveolar ventilation tends to increase; when total ventilation decreases, alveolar ventilation tends to decrease. Because of this rough parallelism, it's common to use the generic term "ventilation" to refer loosely to both total and alveolar ventilation; I sometimes do that in this book.

***Going further**. Technically, minute ventilation is the amount of total ventilation that occurs in one minute. For example, if total ventilation is 7.5 liters/ minute, you'd say that minute ventilation is 7.5 liters, with no mention of "per minute" since that is already included in the definition. However, as a practical matter, the terms total ventilation and minute ventilation are often used interchangeably, usually including "per minute" in both cases.

With that background in place, let's proceed to the subject at hand: the regulation of arterial PCO_2.* The PCO_2 of arterial blood is determined by two main factors: (1) the rate of alveolar ventilation and (2) the rate of CO_2 production by the tissues. Let's look at these individually.

Alveolar Ventilation

Changes in alveolar ventilation cause inverse (opposite direction) changes in arterial PCO_2. When alveolar ventilation increases, arterial PCO_2 decreases. When alveolar ventilation decreases, arterial PCO_2 increases. Think of your own breathing. If you hyperventilate, PCO_2 decreases. Conversely, if you hold your breath—an extreme reduction in ventilation—arterial PCO_2 increases.

These inverse changes make sense physiologically. A higher rate of alveolar ventilation brings more fresh air, which has a low CO_2 content, into the lung's air spaces. The PCO_2 of alveolar air is reduced, which facilitates diffusion of CO_2 out of pulmonary capillary blood, thereby lowering arterial PCO_2. Conversely, when ventilation slows, less fresh air enters the lungs, so the PCO_2 of alveolar air increases. The higher alveolar PCO_2 tends to slow the diffusion of CO_2 out of the pulmonary capillary blood, so arterial PCO_2 rises.

The effects of alveolar ventilation on arterial PCO_2 are not only inverse, they are also proportional, meaning they change by the same percentage degree. For example, if alveolar ventilation doubles, arterial PCO_2 is halved. If alveolar ventilation is halved, arterial PCO_2 doubles. If alveolar ventilation increases by 35 percent, PCO_2 decreases by 35 percent.**

CO_2 Production

If CO_2 production by the tissues increases, arterial PCO_2 tends to increase. If CO_2 production decreases, arterial PCO_2 tends to decrease. I say "tends to" because these changes in PCO_2 occur only if there is no offsetting change in the rate of alveolar ventilation. As you can see, these changes in PCO_2 are direct (same direction), not inverse. Thus, we can say that when ventilation is held constant, arterial PCO_2 changes directly with tissue CO_2 production.

These direct changes also make sense physiologically. When more CO_2 is produced, more enters the blood, so PCO_2 rises. But if ventilation increases at the same time, the lung eliminates CO_2 more efficiently, so arterial PCO_2 doesn't increase. Think of physical exercise: a lot more CO_2 is produced by muscles, but ventilation increases at the same time, so arterial PCO_2 is unchanged. If you exercised but did not increase ventilation, arterial PCO_2 would increase sharply. Conversely, if you sit quietly, CO_2 production will decrease, and your breathing will slow, thus holding arterial PCO_2 constant. However, if you sat quietly and forced yourself to keep breathing at the same rate as when you were active, arterial PCO_2 would decrease.

---

* **Terminology.** Some writers refer to the PCO_2 of arterial blood as $PaCO_2$. I use the simpler term PCO_2 in all cases. The context usually makes clear when I'm speaking about arterial blood.

** **Clinical note.** For example, if a severe asthmatic episode cuts alveolar ventilation in half, PCO_2 can increase to about 80 mm Hg (from a baseline of 40). Conversely, if ventilation doubles due to a panic attack, PCO_2 can fall to 20.

The influence of tissue CO_2 production on arterial PCO_2, like the influence of alveolar ventilation, is proportional, though here the relationship is direct, not inverse. Thus, if CO_2 production rises by 45 percent, PCO_2 will increase by 45 percent—unless alveolar ventilation also increases by 45 percent. As the examples of physical exercise and sitting quietly suggest, alveolar ventilation in a healthy person automatically increases or decreases to match changes in CO_2 production, so arterial PCO_2 is usually stable even when CO_2 production changes markedly.

A Single Formula

The various effects of alveolar ventilation and CO_2 production on arterial PCO_2 can be expressed with a single formula that incorporates the "proportional to" ($\propto$) symbol:

$$\text{Arterial } PCO_2 \propto CO_2 \text{ Production/Alveolar ventilation}$$

To see how this formula works, consider a few examples. When more CO_2 is produced, the numerator increases, causing the value of the fraction to rise—so arterial PCO_2 increases, just as we expect. When alveolar ventilation increases, the denominator increases, causing the value of the fraction to fall—so arterial PCO_2 decreases, again as we expect. The formula also tells you that parallel changes in CO_2 production and alveolar ventilation—say, a 50 percent rise in both CO_2 production and alveolar ventilation—are offsetting and do not change PCO_2. This offset is apparent in the formula since the parallel changes affect the numerator and denominator proportionally and in the same direction, so the value of the fraction is unchanged.

Physiologic Control

In health, the body matches alveolar ventilation to CO_2 production, so arterial PCO_2 stays constant. How does this matching occur? The main mechanism involves feedback from PCO_2-sensitive chemosensors. The most important of these are located in the medulla (the lower portion of the brain stem). The carotid bodies, located near the bifurcation of the common carotid arteries, play a secondary role. The chemosensors are connected via the autonomic nervous system to the respiratory centers in the brain stem, which control the rate and depth (tidal volume) of breathing. When arterial PCO_2 rises, the chemosensors signal for ventilation to increase. When arterial PCO_2 falls, the chemosensors signal for ventilation to decrease. Even small changes in arterial blood PCO_2 are rapidly detected and corrected.*

---

* **Hint.** It's worth emphasizing that it is PCO_2, not PO_2, to which the sensors are primarily responsive. Likewise, it is the elevated arterial PCO_2 that makes you feel starved for air during an extended breath hold. This fact explains why it can be dangerous to hyperventilate before swimming underwater. Hyperventilation, by reducing PCO_2, removes the stimulus to breathe, making it possible to swim without air hunger right until you pass out underwater from lack of oxygen (hypoxia). **Going further.** The PCO_2 chemosensors work, at least in part, by sensing changes in the pH in their immediate fluid environment, including the cerebrospinal fluid and brain interstitial fluid. Because changes in PCO_2 rapidly affect the equilibrium position of the $CO_2 + H_2O \rightleftharpoons H^+ + HCO_3^-$ buffer system, thereby altering pH, pH sensitivity provides a good sensing mechanism for changes in PCO_2.

In addition to these feedback systems, there are also mechanisms that anticipate (or predict) changes in CO_2 production even before there is a chance for PCO_2 to change. For example, during exercise, movement sensors in joints and muscles may signal the respiratory centers to increase ventilation as soon as movement first occurs, thus keeping PCO_2 from rising even slightly.

Summary

CO_2 is produced by the tissues and is carried in venous blood (venous PCO_2 = 45 mm Hg) through the right side of the heart and pulmonary arteries into the lung. As blood passes through the pulmonary capillaries, excess CO_2 diffuses into the alveolar air spaces and is eliminated from the body during normal breathing. Blood leaving the lung (PCO_2 = 40) travels through the left side of the heart and systemic arteries. In the systemic (tissue) capillaries, blood PCO_2 increases by 5 mm Hg due to the diffusion of CO_2 from the tissues, where it is produced by aerobic metabolism. The PCO_2 of arterial blood is directly proportional to the rate of CO_2 production ($\uparrow CO_2$ Production causes $\uparrow PCO_2$) and inversely proportional to the rate of alveolar ventilation ($\uparrow$ Alveolar ventilation causes $\downarrow PCO_2$). Both these relationships are expressed in the following formula:

$$\text{Arterial } PCO_2 \propto CO_2 \text{ Production/Alveolar ventilation}$$

In a healthy person, the body automatically adjusts ventilation (through changes in respiratory rate and/or tidal volume) so that alveolar ventilation closely matches changes in CO_2 production, thereby keeping PCO_2 constant. In some disease states, the matching is impaired, causing PCO_2 to increase (respiratory acidosis) or decrease (respiratory alkalosis). We'll study these disease states in detail in Chapters 8 and 9.

Chapter 4

Acid-Base Physiology: The Kidney

This chapter begins with a brief overview of general renal physiology and then explains how, in healthy persons, the kidneys keep plasma bicarbonate concentration ($[HCO_3^-]$) stable at about 24 mmol/l. As you'll see, the kidneys maintain $[HCO_3^-]$ at this level through the processes of bicarbonate reabsorption and bicarbonate regeneration. Understanding this chapter will give you a strong foundation for studying the metabolic acid-base disorders (i.e., metabolic acidosis and metabolic alkalosis).

Overview of General Renal Physiology

The **nephron** is the functional unit—the working subcomponent—of the kidney. The two kidneys together contain about 1.5 million nephrons. Each nephron carries out nearly all the functions of the kidney as a whole, and each produces a tiny amount of urine every day. Taken together, the urine from these 1.5 million nephrons composes the body's total urine output. Scan this figure of a nephron and refer to it as you continue to read:

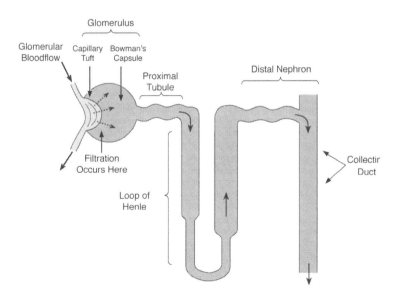

You can picture the nephron as having two main structures: the **glomerulus** (on the upper left of the figure) and a long tubule (literally, "little tube") that extends from the glomerulus. In the above figure, the **tubule** comprises everything but the glomerulus. The glomerulus itself has two main parts: a **capillary tuft** and **Bowman's capsule**. The capillary tuft is a network of capillaries bunched together into a small mass. Blood flows into and out of the tuft via small vessels (shown in the extreme left of the figure). The blood vessel that enters the tuft is a branch of the renal artery; and the vessel that exits the tuft is a tributary of the renal vein. Bowman's capsule, which is the dilated end of the tubule, is pressed tightly against the capillary tuft. The tubule is divided into several main sections: **proximal tubule**, **loop of Henle**, and **distal nephron**. The distal nephron itself has several parts, of which the last part, the **collecting duct**, is the most important for acid-base balance, as you'll see later in the chapter.*

As blood passes through the capillary tuft, some of the fluid from blood plasma is **filtered** from the capillary into Bowman's capsule. This **filtration** process is shown in the figure with dashed arrows. Water and small solutes (sodium, glucose, urea, etc.) are filtered. In contrast, blood cells and platelets, as well as most of the large plasma proteins (e.g., albumin), normally stay behind in the capillaries. Because it enters Bowman's capsule by filtration, fluid in the capsule is known as **filtrate**. Once this fluid passes out of Bowman's capsule into the rest of the tubule, it is referred to simply as **tubular fluid**, since it is located in the tubule proper. The entry of filtrate into Bowman's capsule creates a one-way fluid flow away from the glomerulus. The direction of this fluid flow is shown in the figure above with arrows located inside the tubule.

Although the tubule undergoes twists and turns, it is a hollow tube throughout. Thus, a cross section at any point along the tubule's length is roughly circular. Study this tubular cross section for a moment, then refer back to it as you continue reading:

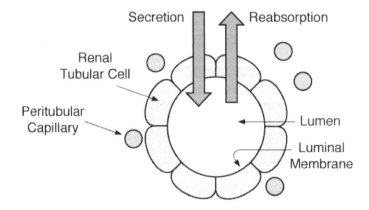

Start by noticing that the tubule wall consists of a single layer of cells. These cells are known as **renal tubular cells** or, more simply, **tubular cells**. The central space of the tubule is called the **lumen**. Thus, the tubular fluid (which is found in the lumen) can also be called **luminal fluid**. The inner surface of the tubule, which

---

* **Terminology**. In the nephron, proximal and distal are defined with respect to the glomerulus. Proximal = "close to" the glomerulus. Distal = "remote from" the glomerulus. The first part of the collecting duct is sometimes called the collecting tubule, but since the general term collecting duct encompasses both the collecting tubule and the rest of the collecting duct system, I'll use the term "collecting duct" in all cases.

faces the lumen, is called the luminal surface or the **luminal membrane**. Notice that capillaries run along the outside of the tubule. These capillaries are shown here as small circles because they are being viewed in cross section, like the tubule itself. Because these capillaries are located around the tubule, they are sometimes called **peritubular capillaries** (peritubular = "around the tubule") to distinguish them from the glomerular capillaries (i.e., the capillaries that make up the glomerular capillary tuft).*

Continuing with the same figure, focus on the large arrows labeled "secretion" and "reabsorption." **Secretion** refers to the transport of substances into the tubular fluid. It provides a second route (in addition to filtration) for substances to enter the lumen. Secretion is essential because it allows the kidneys to eliminate particular substances from the body more rapidly and selectively than would be possible by filtration alone. **Reabsorption** refers to the transport of substances out of the tubular fluid. Reabsorption is essential because more water and solutes are filtered than can safely leave the body. Without reabsorption, normal filtration would rapidly cause a life-threatening depletion of water and electrolytes (ions). Secretion and reabsorption are carried out by renal tubular cells. Most substances that are secreted come from blood in the peritubular capillaries, and most substances that are reabsorbed enter blood in the peritubular capillaries. This peritubular blood enters the kidney via the renal artery, and it exits the kidney via the renal vein and returns to the main systemic circulation. As a result, reabsorbed substances are distributed to extracellular fluid (ECF) throughout the body.

Where does **urine** fit in? As filtrate travels down the tubule—from proximal tubule, to loop of Henle, to distal nephron—it is repeatedly subject to reabsorption and secretion, with each nephron segment reabsorbing and secreting particular substances. Urine is what is left at the end of the process, after all reabsorption and secretion has taken place. Put differently, it is reabsorption and secretion that turns filtrate into urine. In fact, you can define urine like this:

Urine = material filtered − material reabsorbed + material secreted

Urine from all the collecting ducts in each kidney combines and flows together into the renal pelvis, a hollow area in the center of the kidney. From the pelvis, urine travels down the ureter, into the bladder, and is ultimately **excreted** from the body. Note that excretion is defined as elimination from the body. Don't confuse excretion with secretion. Secretion refers to the transport of materials into the tubular lumen, not to excretion from the body. Secretion helps create urine, which is ultimately excreted, but secretion is not itself a process of excretion.

Each day, well over 100 liters of filtrate enter the kidneys' tubules. To describe the rate of filtration, the term **glomerular filtration rate (GFR)** is used. The "classic"

---

* **Hint**. In the figure on page 37, the peritubular capillaries are not shown because I wanted to keep that figure as clear and simple as possible. If we added peritubular capillaries to that figure, they would extend along the length of the tubule, either running more-or-less parallel to the tubule or forming a network around it, a bit like a fish-net stocking around a very thin leg.

value for GFR is often said to be 180 liters per day, but in reality there is much person-to-person variation, with average values ranging from about 135 to 180 liters per day. (GFR varies markedly depending on body size, lean muscle mass, and other factors.). Almost all of this filtered fluid is reabsorbed, so only about one liter of actual urine is produced and excreted each day.

With that background in place, let's now move on to the main subject of this chapter.

Bicarbonate Reabsorption and Regeneration

Assuming a GFR of 180 liters per day and a normal plasma $[HCO_3^-]$ of 24 mmol/l, approximately 4,320 millimoles (i.e., 180 x 24) of bicarbonate are filtered from blood into the renal tubules each day. To keep plasma $[HCO_3^-]$ from falling, this large quantity of filtered bicarbonate must be returned to the blood—that is, it must be reabsorbed. This process is called **bicarbonate reabsorption**. As mentioned above, reabsorption is carried out by renal tubular cells, and the reabsorption of bicarbonate is no exception.

Bicarbonate reabsorption is essential but, by itself, it cannot keep plasma $[HCO_3^-]$ from falling. Here's why. As part of its normal functioning, the body continually produces small amounts of strong acid. This acid is released into the body's internal fluids. For example, the metabolism of sulfur-containing amino acids from food in the diet generates sulfuric acid. Other bodily processes produce strong acids as well. Taken together, all of the body's strong-acid producing processes are referred to as **endogenous acid production (EAP)**. Endogenous acids, being strong acids, dissociate fully, releasing protons. These protons are buffered by plasma bicarbonate via the reaction $H^+ + HCO_3^- \rightarrow CO_2 + H_2O$. This reaction consumes (uses up) bicarbonate.* If this lost bicarbonate is not replaced, $[HCO_3^-]$ in the ECF will gradually fall, causing metabolic acidosis. The kidneys carry out this replacement of bicarbonate by a process called **bicarbonate regeneration**, so named because it regenerates lost bicarbonate. A typical rate of endogenous acid production in a healthy individual produces about 70 millimoles (mmols) of H^+ per day, which consumes about 70 mmols of bicarbonate—so about 70 mmols of bicarbonate must be regenerated each day.

Thus, it is the *combination* of bicarbonate reabsorption (which returns filtered bicarbonate to the blood) and bicarbonate regeneration (which replaces bicarbonate that is lost while buffering endogenously produced strong acids) that keeps plasma $[HCO_3^-]$ stable. Bicarbonate regeneration, like bicarbonate reabsorption, is carried out by renal tubular cells. If reabsorption is 100 percent complete *and* some bicarbonate regeneration also occurs, $[HCO_3^-]$ in the renal vein will be very slightly *higher* than in the renal artery.

---

* **Hint**. As a reminder, the CO_2 produced by this buffering reaction enters the blood, is carried to the lung, and is eliminated in exhaled air along with the much larger amount of CO_2 produced by normal tissue metabolism. The tiny amount of water produced by the buffering reaction (typically about 1 ml per day) enters the body's fluid pool.

Bicarbonate regeneration occurs through two different processes: **ammonium excretion** and **titratable acid excretion**—and we'll study the details of both shortly. Since ammonium excretion and titratable acid excretion are the only two routes by which the kidneys regenerate bicarbonate, you can write a simple equation like this:

Bicarbonate regeneration = Ammonium excretion + Titratable acid excretion

This equation indicates that the sum of bicarbonate regenerated by ammonium excretion and titratable acid excretion equals total regenerated bicarbonate. As its name suggests, ammonium excretion results in the appearance of **ammonium (NH_4^+)** in the urine. Likewise, titratable acid excretion results in the appearance of **titratable acids** (a term I'll comment on later) in the urine. So, in overview, there are three bicarbonate-handling processes that are carried out by renal tubular cells: bicarbonate reabsorption, ammonium excretion, and titratable acid excretion—with the last two accounting for bicarbonate regeneration.

These three bicarbonate-handling processes have a great deal in common. Most importantly, all involve **proton secretion**—that is, the secretion of protons by the renal tubular cells into the tubular lumen. Therefore, before looking at each bicarbonate-handling process individually, it's useful to study proton secretion by itself. Start by studying the following figure of a renal tubular cell. Try to visualize the cell as one among many in the more-or-less cylindrical wall of the tubule, consistent with the cross-sectional figure on page 38. Then keep reading, referring back to the figure as you go.

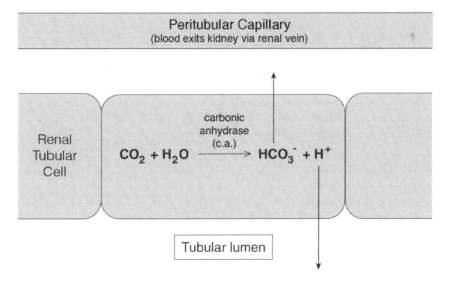

Notice that inside the renal tubular cell, protons (H^+) are produced by the reaction $CO_2 + H_2O \rightarrow HCO_3^- + H^+$. Both CO_2 and H_2O are ubiquitous in the body fluids, including inside cells, so there is no shortage of these reactants. The reaction is catalyzed by the enzyme carbonic anhydrase. The newly produced H^+

is secreted into the lumen, where it acidifies (lowers the pH of) the tubular fluid. Now, notice that proton secretion does not occur in isolation. The same reaction that produced the proton ($CO_2 + H_2O \rightarrow HCO_3^- + H^+$) also produces bicarbonate, HCO_3^-. This newly produced HCO_3^- is transported in the opposite direction from the proton; it enters the blood of a peritubular capillary, which leaves the kidney via the renal vein. Since protons and bicarbonate are produced in a 1:1 ratio, one bicarbonate enters the blood for each proton that is secreted into the nephron lumen. We can even say that the secretion of H^+ into the lumen and the entry of HCO_3^- into the blood represent two aspects of the same cellular process, or two sides of the same coin. This is a key point. Make sure you understand it clearly.

These steps involving protons and bicarbonate occur in each of the three bicarbonate-handling processes (bicarbonate reabsorption, ammonium excretion, and titratable acid excretion). *The main difference among the three processes is what happens to the secreted proton once it enters the lumen.* This point will become clear as you continue to read. Let's now study the three bicarbonate-handling processes individually.*

Bicarbonate Reabsorption

Start by scanning this figure:

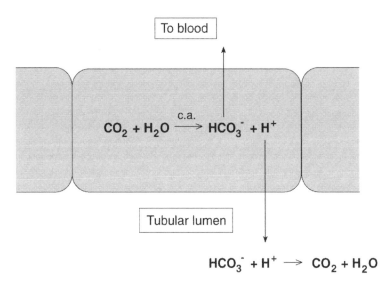

This figure reproduces the one just shown but adds a new element: the secreted H^+ gets buffered in the lumen by combining with bicarbonate in the tubular fluid via the reaction $HCO_3^- + H^+ \rightarrow CO_2 + H_2O$. (This reaction is the exact opposite of the one, inside the cell, that produced the proton in the first place.) This luminal bicarbonate got into the lumen by filtration. Notice that when the luminal bicarbonate ion combines with the secreted proton, the bicarbonate

---

* **Looking Ahead**. You may have noticed that I did not describe the molecular transporters that actually carry the protons across the cell membrane into the lumen. We'll study those transporters in the final section of this chapter (pages. 48–50), after you have a good grasp of the overall processes.

"disappears"; it is converted to CO_2 and water. At the same time, a completely different bicarbonate ion, produced inside the cell, enters the blood of the peritubular capillary. The net result is that a filtered bicarbonate ion disappears from the lumen and (in effect) reappears in the blood. This result is *exactly the same as would have happened if bicarbonate had been directly transported from the lumen to the blood.* However, direct lumen-to-blood bicarbonate transport does not occur.

The overall process I just described is what is referred to as bicarbonate reabsorption. As you can see, this use of the term "reabsorption" is slightly unconventional, because reabsorption in the usual sense (the transport of a molecule or ion from lumen to blood) does not occur for bicarbonate. But because the net effect of the process (a bicarbonate ion disappears from the lumen and appears in the blood) is the same as would have occurred with direct reabsorption, the term bicarbonate reabsorption is still used.*

About 85 percent of filtered bicarbonate is reabsorbed in the proximal tubule. Of the remaining 15 percent, about half is reabsorbed in the loop of Henle and half is reabsorbed in the distal nephron. (Glance back to the figure on page 37 if you need a reminder of where these structures are located.)

Ammonium Excretion

Once again, start by scanning this figure:

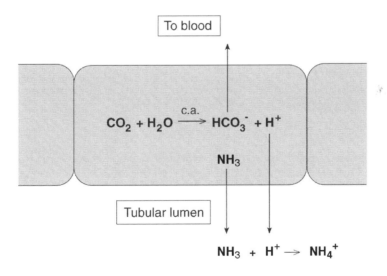

* **Hint.** If you find it easier to imagine, as a mental shorthand, that actual reabsorption does occur, no harm is done since the consequences are the same. To see even more clearly that the consequences are identical, consider what happens if reabsorption fails. First, bicarbonate that is filtered at the glomerulus is not replaced in the blood, so plasma $[HCO_3^-]$ falls. Second, bicarbonate remains in the nephron lumen and eventually appears in the urine, and the amount of bicarbonate in the urine precisely equals the amount of bicarbonate lost from blood during filtration. These same two outcomes would occur regardless of whether one assumes a failure of actual reabsorption or a failure of the reabsorption-like process that occurs in reality.

Here, everything is the same as before except that the secreted proton, instead of combining with bicarbonate, combines with **ammonia (NH$_3$)**, forming ammonium (NH$_4^+$).* The NH$_3$ comes from inside renal tubular cells. It crosses the luminal membrane in parallel with the secreted proton, as shown. The ammonia is derived from the amino acid glutamine. This glutamine is metabolized inside renal tubular cells and its two nitrogen-containing groups are split off, forming ammonia. This figure shows the structure of glutamine, with the nitrogen groups marked:

$$NH_3$$

$$NH_3^+$$

$$H - C - CH_2 - CH_2 - C + NH_2 \qquad NH_3$$

$$\overset{O}{\overset{\|}{C}}$$

$$COO^-$$

Ammonia (NH$_3$) is a strong base, so it readily combines with secreted protons. As in bicarbonate reabsorption, each secreted proton is associated with the entry of one bicarbonate into the blood. Be sure to notice that in the figure. Since the secreted proton combines with ammonia, and the resulting ammonium ends up in the urine, you can quantify the entire process by measuring urinary ammonium. That is, each ammonium in the urine indicates the addition of one new bicarbonate to the blood. Once again, be sure you understand this point from the figure.

All this looks quite similar to bicarbonate reabsorption, and it is. But a key difference is that in ammonium excretion the newly produced bicarbonate is not merely a replacement for a filtered bicarbonate ion, as occurs during bicarbonate reabsorption. Rather, the new bicarbonate can actually increase the [HCO$_3^-$] of the body fluids, raising plasma [HCO$_3^-$] back to normal if it should fall for any reason. It is this aspect of the process—the ability to raise plasma [HCO$_3^-$] above its current level—that causes the process to be described as bicarbonate regeneration: that is, the process *regenerates* lost bicarbonate. Because luminal buffering by ammonia occurs mostly in the collecting duct, ammonium excretion is usually said to be a distal process.**

---

* **Mnemonic**. If you tend to confuse ammonia (NH$_3$) and ammonium (NH$_4^+$), look at the last three letters of "ammonium" and let your eyes blur. With a little imagination, you'll see the word "ion." Ammonium is an ion; ammonia is not.

** **Going further.** Ammonium excretion is a complex process, which I have simplified somewhat to ensure that the main points are clear. In reality, ammonium excretion is not entirely a distal process, in that most glutamine actually gets metabolized inside the cells of the proximal tubule. From there, ammonia (as well as some ammonium) travels to the distal tubular cells via, among other things, a counter-current multiplier in the interstitium of the kidney. Understanding these fine points is not important for our purposes and I won't say more about them.

Titratable Acid Excretion

As before, scan this figure, then keep reading:

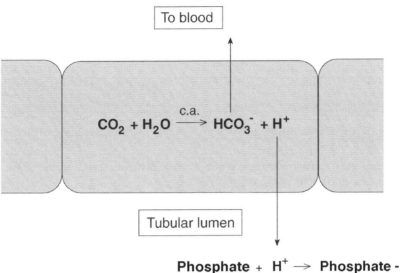

In this figure, everything is the same as before except that here the secreted proton combines with phosphate.* Most of the phosphate in the lumen gets there by filtration. Notice that each proton that combines with a filtered phosphate is matched by a newly produced bicarbonate added to the blood. As in ammonium excretion, this newly produced bicarbonate can actually increase plasma $[HCO_3^-]$, replacing lost bicarbonate in the body fluids. Thus, like ammonium excretion, titratable acid excretion is considered a form of bicarbonate regeneration.

In addition to phosphate, there are several other non-bicarbonate substances in the tubular fluid that can accept protons, act as buffers, and thus contribute to titratable acid excretion. These include urate and creatinine. However, these substances usually are present in lower quantities than phosphate and are not as good buffers (their pK is further from the pH of luminal fluid), so their contribution is usually small. As a practical matter, you can disregard them.

Once phosphate and the other non-bicarbonate urinary buffers are protonated in the nephron lumen, they are referred to as **titratable acids**—hence the name titratable acid excretion.** Titratable acid excretion occurs in both the proximal

---

* **Going further**. Phosphate has different forms, depending on how many protons it has—no protons (PO_4^{3-}), monoprotic (HPO_4^{2-}), diprotic ($H_2PO_4^{1-}$), and triprotic (H_3PO_4). The equilibrium between monoprotic and diprotic phosphate ($HPO_4^{2-} + H^+ \rightleftharpoons H_2PO_4^{1-}$) has a pK of 6.8, making it a good buffer in both blood and urine. Monoprotic phosphate is the primary proton acceptor during titratable acid excretion.

** **Terminology**. The name "titratable acid" is used because a special titration assay, performed on urine, can determine the quantity of protons that were buffered by these substances. This assay is rarely done now—it is mostly of historical importance—but I mention it to give you a sense of where the unusual name "titratable acid" comes from.

and distal nephron (collecting duct). In most circumstances, these two locations produce about equal amounts of titratable acid and, hence, equal amounts of new bicarbonate.

Let's summarize key points. Bicarbonate reabsorption (which is not reabsorption in the usual sense), ammonium (NH_4^+) excretion, and titratable acid (T.A.) excretion all are built on the process of proton secretion. The main difference is that the secreted H^+ combines with different buffers in the lumen. In bicarbonate reabsorption, the H^+ combines with filtered bicarbonate, causing that filtered bicarbonate to "disappear"; in ammonium excretion, the H^+ combines with ammonia (NH_3), forming ammonium (NH_4^+); in T.A. excretion, the H^+ combines with filtered phosphate (and a few other minor buffers), forming "titratable acid." Whereas reabsorption of bicarbonate replaces bicarbonate lost from the blood during filtration, excretion of NH_4^+ and T.A. regenerates, and thus replaces, bicarbonate lost during the buffering of endogenously produced strong acids. By replacing both the bicarbonate lost during filtration and the bicarbonate lost during buffering of endogenously produced acids, the combination of bicarbonate reabsorption and bicarbonate regeneration can keep plasma [HCO_3^-] stable.

Bicarbonate Balance in the Body

Let's now focus on the big picture: a bird's eye view of bicarbonate gains and losses in the body. I'll start with a few words about terminology. Ammonium (NH_4^+) is the conjugate acid (i.e., the protonated form) of ammonia (NH_3), which functions as a base (proton acceptor). Likewise, the titratable acids (T.A.) are the conjugate acids of bases such as phosphate. This means that you can broadly categorize NH_4^+ and T.A. as acids. For this reason, the sum of NH_4^+ excretion and T.A. excretion is sometimes simply termed "acid excretion." As we've seen, this sum is itself equal to bicarbonate regeneration. Putting all this together:

Acid excretion = NH_4^+ excretion + T.A. excretion = Bicarbonate regeneration

To this point in the chapter, I've been writing as if all filtered bicarbonate is re-absorbed. In reality, there is a very slight inefficiency in the process. Even when the kidneys are functioning well, a few mmols per day of bicarbonate fail to be reabsorbed. This unreabsorbed bicarbonate, which appears in the urine, is lost from the body. Therefore, if we want to understand the net bicarbonate contribution of the kidney (by net, I mean gains minus losses), and hence the kidney's overall effect on plasma [HCO_3^-], we have to subtract urinary bicarbonate (bicarbonate lost from the body) from bicarbonate regeneration (bicarbonate gained by the body). That is, we subtract urinary bicarbonate from the sum of urinary ammonium and titratable acids. The difference is **net bicarbonate regeneration**. Because ammonium and titratable acid are acids, and bicarbonate is a base, we can also think of this quantity as acid minus base, and we can describe it as **net acid excretion (NAE)**:

NAE = Urinary ammonium + Urinary titratable acid – Urinary bicarbonate

Here's an example. If, during a 24-hour period, ammonium excretion is 40 mmols, titratable acid excretion is 35 mmols, and urinary bicarbonate spillage is 2 mmols, then NAE is 73 mmols (40 + 35 − 2). The kidney has added 73 mmols of bicarbonate to the blood. Put differently, over the 24 hours in question, blood leaving the kidneys in the renal veins has 73 mmols more bicarbonate than blood entering the kidneys in the renal arteries.

As I mentioned before (p. 40), the total amount of strong acid that is produced in the body is termed endogenous acid production. The protons released from this acid are buffered by bicarbonate. To keep the body's total bicarbonate stores (and hence plasma $[HCO_3^-]$) from decreasing, net acid excretion, and hence net bicarbonate regeneration, is regulated to match endogenous acid production, like this:

Net acid excretion (NAE) = Endogenous acid excretion (EAP)

Maintaining this equality—through the tight regulation of NAE by the kidney—keeps the body in balance for bicarbonate and hence keeps $[HCO_3^-]$ stable. Maintaining this balance is the overall acid-base task of the kidney.* In a healthy individual, ammonium excretion and titratable acid excretion are roughly equal (about 35 mmols/day each). But during metabolic acidosis, when bicarbonate regeneration is maximally stimulated to replace the large amount of bicarbonate that is lost, ammonium excretion becomes more important because the kidney can increase ammonium excretion by up to ten times. This increase in ammonium excretion is homeostatic ("tending to reestablish a normal state") because it minimizes further declines in plasma $[HCO_3^-]$ and, ultimately, helps restore plasma $[HCO_3^-]$ to normal. In contrast, the body does not have a way to homeostatically increase titratable acid excretion, so the rate is usually fairly constant.

The following table summarizes some key features of renal bicarbonate handling. It highlights the similarities among bicarbonate reabsorption, bicarbonate regeneration, and titratable acid excretion. Take a moment to study this table, to be sure it all makes sense to you, before continuing.

---

* **Going further**. These statements presume that all EAP is buffered by bicarbonate. What about non-bicarbonate buffers, such as hemoglobin and plasma proteins? Some protons from EAP are, in fact, buffered by these non-bicarbonate buffers. However, as bicarbonate is regenerated by the kidney, plasma $[HCO_3^-]$ rises slightly; the resulting rise in pH shifts the equilibrium points of the non-bicarbonate buffers, causing them to release protons, which then combine with and consume additional bicarbonate. Thus, the non-bicarbonate buffers serve merely as temporary storage sites for protons, not as permanent removal mechanisms; all protons (except for a trivial amount of free H^+) are ultimately buffered and removed by bicarbonate. In bookkeeping terms, when calculating bicarbonate balance, it's as if the non-bicarbonate buffers didn't even exist.

	Bicarbonate Reabsorption	Bicarbonate Regeneration	
		Titratable acid excretion	Ammonium Excretion
Source of bicarbonate that enters the blood	Reaction inside renal tubular cells: $CO_2 + H_2O \rightarrow HCO_3^- + H^+$	Reaction inside renal tubular cells: $CO_2 + H_2O \rightarrow HCO_3^- + H^+$	Reaction inside renal tubular cells: $CO_2 + H_2O \rightarrow HCO_3^- + H^+$
Disposal of protons	Secreted into nephron lumen.	Secreted into nephron lumen.	Secreted into nephron lumen.
What happens to protons in the lumen	Combine with filtered bicarbonate: $H^+ + HCO_3^- \rightarrow CO_2 + H_2O$.	Combine with filtered non-bicarbonate buffers, especially phosphate.	Combine with NH_3 that enters lumen from renal cells: $H^+ + NH_3 \rightarrow NH_4^+$
Quantity of bicarbonate that enters the blood	Almost equal to filtered bicarbonate load. Just a few mmol bicarbonate lost in urine each day.	Roughly 35 mmol/day in most circumstances.	Roughly 35 mmol/day. Can increase ten fold during metabolic acidosis.
Location in nephron	About 85% in proximal tubule. The rest occurs in the loop of Henle and distal nephron.	Both proximal tubule and distal nephron.	Protons secreted and combine with NH_3 mostly in the distal nephron.

Summary of Bicarbonate Handling

Mechanisms of Proton Secretion

A few pages ago, we looked at simple illustrations of renal tubular cells carrying out their bicarbonate-handling functions (pages 41–43). In those figures, I showed proton secretion with arrows but didn't indicate how that secretion occurs. In this final part of the chapter, we'll briefly study the cellular mechanisms involved. As you'll see, there are two main mechanisms of proton secretion, with a third that becomes important in a particular circumstance. Start by studying this figure—then keep reading:

Proximal Tuble   Collecting Duct

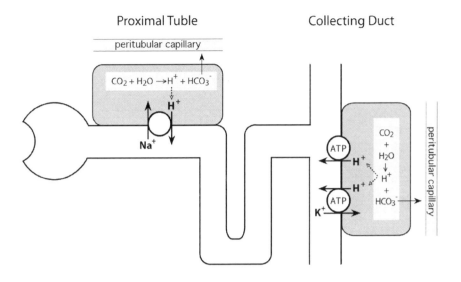

Here we see a highly simplified nephron with just two renal tubular cells—one proximal (left), one distal (right). These cells are drawn disproportionately large for clarity; in reality, there are numerous, small cells that form a thin layer surrounding the lumen. These are the same cell types shown in the earlier figures, but here I've located them along the nephron and added proton transport mechanisms. Before reading about the details, pause to notice two main themes, both of which we've touched on already. First, the cells are localized to two main areas: the proximal tubule and the collecting duct portion of the distal nephron. These are the areas where most of the kidney's main acid-base operations (proton secretion, bicarbonate handling) take place. Second, as you saw in the earlier figures, notice again that protons and bicarbonate are simultaneously produced inside cells by the reaction $CO_2 + H_2O \rightarrow HCO_3^- + H^+$. The result is that every time a proton is secreted into the lumen, a bicarbonate ion leaves the cell in the opposite direction and enters the blood. Let's now examine the proton-secreting mechanisms in detail. Refer to the above figure as you read.

In the cell on the left (proximal tubular cell) a proton moves across the luminal membrane in exchange for Na^+. This process occurs via an **Na^+–H^+ exchanger**. The Na^+ naturally moves into the cell because the luminal fluid has a high $[Na^+]$ (about the same as that of blood plasma, roughly 140 mmol/l) whereas the intracellular fluid has a low $[Na^+]$ (about 1/10th that of plasma). It is this "downhill"—higher to lower concentration—movement of Na^+ into cells that drives proton secretion.* Most Na^+–H^+ exchangers are located in the proximal tubule. Remember

---

* **Hint**. In thinking about how Na^+ and H^+ movements are linked, I like the simple image of water flowing downhill and driving gears on a mill. In this analogy, water is like Na^+ (both flow "downhill") and the gears on the mill are like the proteins in the Na^+–H^+ exchanger that propel H^+ into the lumen. What creates the downhill concentration gradient? Luminal $[Na^+]$ is relatively high, about the same as that of plasma, because luminal fluid is created from plasma by filtration. Intracellular $[Na^+]$ is low because the cell's Na^+–K^+–ATPase transporters continuously transport Na^+ out of the cell.

that about 85 percent of filtered bicarbonate is reabsorbed proximally. It is these Na^+-H^+ exchangers that do most of the proton secretion during proximal tubule bicarbonate reabsorption. These same proximal Na^+-H^+ exchangers also secrete the protons used to form titratable acids in the proximal tubule.

Continuing with the figure, focus now on the cell to the right, which is located in the collecting duct. Here we see two different proton-secreting mechanisms in the same cell. The top mechanism is known as either an **H^+–ATPase** or a **proton pump**. As the (first) name suggests, this pump requires energy in the form of ATP. The special characteristic of the proton pump is that it can secrete protons against a steep gradient—that is, into areas of very high $[H^+]$. It is this characteristic of the proton pumps that lets the collecting duct produce luminal fluid, and hence urine, with a pH as low as 4.4. In contrast, the proximal Na^+-H^+ exchanger can lower pH only to around 6.8. It is the distal proton pumps that secrete most of the protons that are used in ammonium excretion. These same proton pumps also secrete protons used in distal bicarbonate reabsorption and titratable acid excretion.

The last proton secreting mechanism shown is called either an **H^+-K^+ exchanger** or an **H^+-K^+–ATPase**. It secretes an H^+ in exchange for a K^+, which is reabsorbed from the lumen. Like the proton pump, this exchanger is powered by ATP. However, unlike the proton pump, the H^+-K^+ exchanger usually plays a very minor role in H^+ secretion. Only during hypokalemia (low plasma $[K^+]$), when distal K^+ reabsorption is stimulated to help prevent additional K^+ from being lost in the urine, does the exchanger become an important contributor to proton secretion.

One final detail: There are several different types of cells in the collecting duct. The particular kind of cell shown in the figure is called an **alpha-intercalated cell** (a.k.a. A-type intercalated cell). These cells are home to the proton-secreting H^+–ATPase as well as many of the H^+-K^+ exchangers. It is these cells that carry out almost all proton secretion in the distal nephron.

Summary

The renal tubule carries out two main acid-base functions: (1) it reabsorbs almost all filtered bicarbonate and (2) it regenerates new bicarbonate to replace bicarbonate that is lost buffering endogenously produced strong acids. Two processes account for bicarbonate regeneration: ammonium (NH_4^+) excretion and titratable acid (T.A.) excretion. Ammonium excretion is more important because it can homeostatically increase up to ten times when more bicarbonate is needed, as in metabolic acidosis. Bicarbonate reabsorption, NH_4^+ excretion, and T.A. excretion all produce bicarbonate and protons inside renal tubular cells through the reaction $CO_2 + H_2O \rightarrow HCO_3^- + H^+$. Bicarbonate from this reaction enters the blood whereas the protons are secreted into the nephron lumen. In bicarbonate reabsorption, the secreted protons combine with filtered bicarbonate; in T.A. excretion, the secreted protons combine mostly with filtered phosphate; in NH_4^+ excretion, the secreted protons combine with ammonia (NH_3), which is converted to ammonium (NH_4^+). Protons are secreted by three mechanisms: $Na^+–H^+$ exchange (proximal tubule), proton pumps—a.k.a. $H^+–ATPase$ (collecting duct, in distal nephron), and $H^+–K^+$ exchange (collecting duct, in distal nephron; important only during hypokalemia).

Overview to This Point in the Book

Since we're about to shift our focus from physiology to clinical acid-base, this is a good time to summarize the main themes of the book so far, using a single illustration. Spend a moment studying this figure before starting Chapter 5.

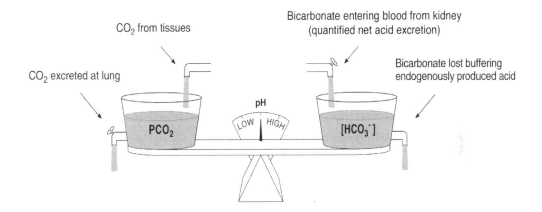

Compensation: A "Damage Limitation" Strategy

In this chapter, which forms the transition to the clinical part of this book, we look at the process of **compensation**. As you'll see, the term compensation refers to a strategy the body uses to help stabilize pH when an acid-base disturbance occurs. Buffering helps stabilize pH, too, and in this sense buffering is also a "damage limitation" strategy. However, in contrast to buffering, which occurs almost instantaneously and is *chemical* in nature, compensation occurs gradually and is *physiological* in nature, meaning that it arises from the action of organs. This distinction will become clear as you proceed. The material in this chapter is important for its own sake and it also provides an essential foundation for interpreting arterial blood gases, which we study in Chapter 11. Start by looking (once again) at this balance figure:

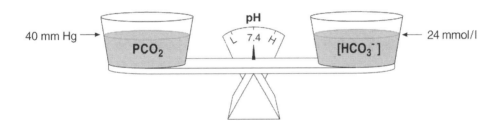

Using this figure as a guide, remind yourself how changes in PCO_2 and $[HCO_3^-]$ affect pH. Use your imagination to double or halve PCO_2 and see which way the scale tips. Do the same for $[HCO_3^-]$. Now try something new. In your mind's eye, double *both* PCO_2 and $[HCO_3^-]$ at the same time. Then reset the scale and halve *both* PCO_2 and $[HCO_3^-]$ at the same time. What happens to pH in these situations? These proportional changes in PCO_2 and $[HCO_3^-]$ keep the scale in balance, so pH does not change. Mathematically, we can say that pH is determined not by PCO_2 or $[HCO_3^-]$ alone, but by the ratio between them. If the ratio doesn't change, pH won't change either.

Now try this. Double PCO_2 and increase—but don't quite double—$[HCO_3^-]$. What happens to pH? If you're visualizing well, you'll see that pH decreases, but not nearly as much as it would have had you'd left $[HCO_3^-]$ unchanged. Now reset the scale and try this: halve PCO_2 and reduce—but don't quite halve—$[HCO_3^-]$. What happens to pH? Here, pH increases, but not nearly as much as it would have had you'd left $[HCO_3^-]$ unchanged. From these visualizations, you can infer this general rule: *If you change one variable (either PCO_2 or $[HCO_3^-]$), you can minimize the change in pH by moving the other variable in the same direction.*

The body makes use of this general rule during the process of compensation. If a pathologic change in either $[HCO_3^-]$ or PCO_2 occurs, the body automatically responds by bringing about a *same-direction* change in the other variable. This change minimizes the deviation in pH. For example, during metabolic acidosis (low $[HCO_3^-]$), the body responds by increasing alveolar ventilation and hence reducing PCO_2—so both $[HCO_3^-]$ and PCO_2 are low. During respiratory acidosis (elevated PCO_2), the kidney acts to increase plasma $[HCO_3^-]$—so both $[HCO_3^-]$ and PCO_2 are high. In these situations, the original or pathologic change in either PCO_2 or HCO_3^- is sometimes referred to as the **primary change**, since it happens first in the sequence of events. The homeostatic change that occurs in the other variable—which tends to normalize pH—is referred to as **compensatory**, because it tends to counterbalance, or compensate for, the pH change produced by the primary abnormality. The compensatory change can also be called the **secondary change**, because it happens second in the sequence of events, that is, after and in response to the primary change.*

Recap

- Compensation is an automatic, homeostatic response to primary abnormalities in PCO_2 or $[HCO_3^-]$.
- Compensation brings about a same-direction change in the "other" variable.
- Compensation returns pH toward normal.

Compensatory changes occur because the primary (pathologic) change in $[HCO_3^-]$ or PCO_2 is sensed and responded to by the organ that regulates the "other" variable. During metabolic disturbances (defined as a primary change in $[HCO_3^-]$), the respiratory center senses the abnormal $[HCO_3^-]$ and changes the rate of ventilation, altering PCO_2. During respiratory disturbances (defined as a primary change in PCO_2), the kidney senses the altered PCO_2 and changes the rates of bicarbonate regeneration and reabsorption, altering $[HCO_3^-]$.

The following table summarizes much of the above:

** **Terminology.** Using the term *primary* to refer to the initial, pathologic change in either $[HCO_3^-]$ or PCO_2 is closely related to the usage of *primary* introduced in Chapter 2, where we learned about the four *primary acid-base disturbances*. Notice that each of the four primary disturbances consists of a "primary" change in either $[HCO_3^-]$ or PCO_2.*

Disturbance	Pathological Change	Compensatory Change
	This is the original change produced by the disturbance. This change causes pH to deviate from normal. Because this change occurs first in the sequence of events—that is, before compensation—it is often called the primary change.	This is the homeostatic change that the body enacts to return pH towards normal. This change occurs after the onset of, and in response to, the primary change. For this reason, it is sometimes called the secondary change.
Metabolic acidosis	$[HCO_3^-] \downarrow$	$PCO_2 \downarrow$
Metabolic alkalosis	$[HCO_3^-] \uparrow$	$PCO_2 \uparrow$
Respiratory acidosis	$PCO_2 \uparrow$	$[HCO_3^-] \uparrow$
Respiratory alkalosis	$PCO_2 \downarrow$	$[HCO_3^-] \downarrow$

Notice in this table that the compensatory change always moves in the same direction as the primary change. We can thus say that compensation follows the **same-direction rule**. This "rule" must be true because only a same-direction change will return the ratio of $[HCO_3^-]$ to PCO_2, and hence pH, towards their normal values. In contrast, an opposite-direction change would perturb the ratio further and exacerbate the pH abnormality.

Naming the Compensatory Responses

Compensatory changes in $[HCO_3^-]$ are termed either "metabolic" (because they involve bicarbonate) or "renal" (because the kidney brings about the change). For example, the phrases "*renal* compensation for respiratory acidosis" and "*metabolic* compensation for respiratory acidosis" both refer to the secondary rise in plasma $[HCO_3^-]$ that occurs in response to a primary rise in PCO_2. Compensatory changes in PCO_2 are always called "respiratory"—for example, "respiratory compensation for metabolic alkalosis" or "respiratory compensation for metabolic acidosis." These phrases refer to the secondary change in PCO_2 that occurs in response to a primary change in $[HCO_3^-]$.

Effectiveness of Compensation

If the percentage change in the compensatory variable exactly matched the percentage change in the primary variable (say, a 50 percent decrease in PCO_2 matched by a 50 percent decrease in $[HCO_3^-]$), pH would not change at all. In reality, compensation is not quite so efficient. It would be more typical to see a 50 percent primary change matched by—just to give an illustration—a 40 percent secondary change. As a result, even compensated acid-base disturbances cause *some* change in pH. The following figure illustrates this point, using metabolic alkalosis as an example:

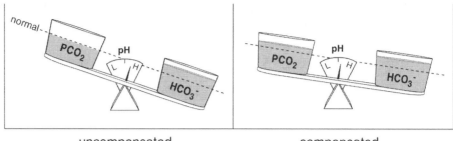

uncompensated   compensated

In general, the compensation for respiratory disturbances is more complete than the compensation for metabolic disturbances. That is, the ratio of $[HCO_3^-]$ to PCO_2 (and hence pH) is closer to normal in compensated respiratory disturbances than in compensated metabolic disturbances. The reason is simply that the mechanisms involved in renal compensation are slightly more efficient than those involved in respiratory compensation. In fact, in some patients with compensated respiratory disturbances, the ratio returns close enough to normal that pH is brought into the normal range (though even in these cases pH does not usually return all the way to the baseline set point for that particular individual). In contrast, in simple metabolic disturbances, pH is always outside the normal range.*

Time for Compensation to Develop

During *metabolic* disturbances, compensatory changes in ventilation begin within 30 minutes, and PCO_2 usually reaches its final compensated level within 12–24 hours. This rapid onset of compensation means that patients with metabolic acidosis or alkalosis are usually partially, or even wholly, compensated by the time they present. Few patients are seen in a totally uncompensated state. In contrast, during *respiratory* disturbances, compensation develops relatively slowly: it usually takes 3–5 days for plasma $[HCO_3^-]$ to reach its final compensated level. Because renal (metabolic) compensation takes relatively long to appear, patients with respiratory acidosis and alkalosis remain in the uncompensated state for a clinically distinct period, and it is not unusual for these patients to present entirely uncompensated. Because distinct uncompensated and compensated states are seen clinically, it is important to differentiate between these two states when referring to respiratory acidosis or alkalosis. One way to do this is with the terms **acute** and **chronic**. In this context, *acute* indicates uncompensated and *chronic* indicates compensated. For example, "He has acute (uncompensated) respiratory acidosis"

***Going further.** It has traditionally been taught that compensation can return pH to the normal range only in respiratory *alkalosis*. However, there is now evidence that some patients with compensated respiratory acidosis can also attain pH values in the normal range, though this question is not fully settled. In this book, I'll presume that both respiratory alkalosis and acidosis, when well compensated, can produce normal-range pH values. Hopefully, new studies will answer the question definitively in time for this book's next edition. In any case, it remains well accepted that pH in simple metabolic disturbances cannot reach the normal range; acidemia or alkalemia are always present unless a mixed disturbance exists.

or "She has chronic (compensated) respiratory alkalosis." Alternatively, you can simply say something like, "He has compensated respiratory acidosis."

Blood Gas Profiles

In Chapter 11, we'll study diagnosis using the arterial blood gas (ABG), which is a test that tells you the pH, PCO_2, and $[HCO_3^-]$ of an arterial blood sample. However, to start you thinking about blood gases, and to reinforce the ideas presented so far in this chapter, let's now look at some ABG profiles. To get oriented, consider this completely normal profile:

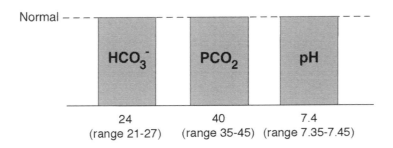

As you can see, I use a single dotted line to indicate the normal levels, even though the three variables have very different normal values. In the profiles that follow, I'll insert some realistic sample values, so you get a sense what the blood gas profile of an actual patient might be. However, keep in mind that the same primary disorder may be more or less severe, so the numbers you encounter in any particular patient may be quite different from those given here.

Metabolic Acidosis

Let's start with metabolic acidosis. Study this figure, then refer back to it as you continue reading:

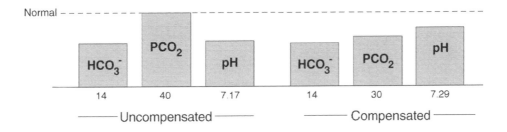

In the uncompensated (left) profile, notice that $[HCO_3^-]$ and (as a result) pH are low, whereas PCO_2 is normal. In the compensated (right) profile, notice three things: (1) the primary change is relatively greater than the secondary (compensatory) change; (2) compensation follows the "same-direction rule"; and (3) compensation minimizes but does not totally eliminate the pH abnormality. These same three points apply to all the primary disturbances. It is important to notice that pH is still somewhat low and outside the normal range. This is as you'd expect for a simple metabolic disturbance, since the compensation for a metabolic disturbance (whether acidosis or alkalosis) does not return pH into the normal range.

Metabolic Alkalosis

The next figure shows metabolic alkalosis. Once again, study the figure, then refer back to it as you continue reading:

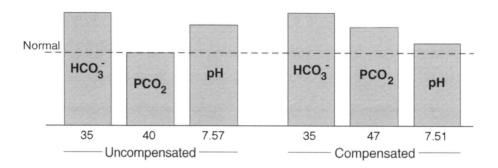

First, look over the uncompensated profile to be sure it makes sense to you. Then, in the compensated profile, notice that pH remains somewhat high and outside the normal range, though it is much closer to normal than in the uncompensated state. This is what you expect for a simple metabolic disturbance.

Respiratory Acidosis

Next, consider respiratory acidosis. Study this figure carefully, and then continue reading.

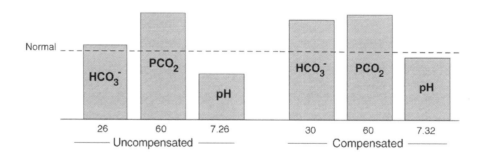

Here there is much to say. First, focus on the uncompensated profile. This patient has "acute respiratory acidosis." This profile reveals something you may not expect. Although compensation has not yet set in, $[HCO_3^-]$ is still slightly above its normal set point. Be sure to notice this in the figure. This small, pre-compensatory rise in $[HCO_3^-]$ occurs because the primary increase in PCO_2 shifts the CO_2 + $H_2O \leftrightharpoons HCO_3^- + H^+$ equilibrium in the ECF slightly to the right, in accordance with Le Chatelier's principle, producing a small amount of additional bicarbonate. (Most of the newly produced protons are buffered by non-bicarbonate buffers such as hemoglobin.) This small equilibrium shift usually leaves $[HCO_3^-]$ within the normal range. Note that this equilibrium shift, and the accompanying rise in $[HCO_3^-]$, occurs *acutely*—it begins instantaneously and is complete within minutes. This acute change is a *chemical* or *buffering* process. That is, it arises as a result of a chemical shift in the bicarbonate buffer equilibrium; plasma $[HCO_3^-]$ rises without the kidney having to regenerate any additional bicarbonate. If you took a beaker of blood and put it into a gas-filled chamber with a high PCO_2, $[HCO_3^-]$ would increase just as it does in the body, and just as quickly.

Now turn your attention to the compensated profile. This patient has "chronic respiratory acidosis." The change in $[HCO_3^-]$ shown here represents the sum of the small, immediate, buffering-related (chemical) change and the large, slower, compensatory change, which is *physiological* in nature. By physiological, I mean it arises from the action of an *organ*. Specifically, it arises from a gradual increase in bicarbonate production (especially via ammonium excretion) by the kidney. As I mentioned, in some patients with chronic respiratory acidosis, pH may be in the normal range. Although the acute (chemical buffering) and chronic (physiological, compensatory) rises in $[HCO_3^-]$ are fundamentally different, they have something important in common: both move $[HCO_3^-]$ in the same direction. That is, both acute and chronic changes follow the same-direction rule.

Respiratory Alkalosis

Finally, consider respiratory alkalosis:

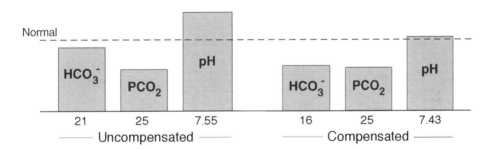

In the uncompensated profile ("acute respiratory alkalosis"), notice the small, pre-compensatory *decline* in $[HCO_3^-]$. This is the reverse of the acute change we just saw in respiratory acidosis. As before, this acute change is nearly instantaneous, chemical in nature, and is due to a shift in the $CO_2 + H_2O \leftrightharpoons HCO_3^- + H^+$ equilibrium that results from the primary change in PCO_2. This time, the shift is to the left and occurs in response to the primary decline in PCO_2. As before, this rapid change typically leaves $[HCO_3^-]$ within the normal range.

Turning to the compensated profile ("chronic respiratory alkalosis"), notice that here—finally!—we see pH is in the normal range. This profile is consistent with the classic teaching that compensated respiratory alkalosis can return pH to the normal range. However, keep in mind that not all patients with chronic respiratory alkalosis will have normal pH values and, even when they do, pH is high-normal. That is, pH does not move all the way to its initial set point (which, for simplicity, I'll assume is 7.40, the mid-point of the normal range). Finally, let me again emphasize the distinction between the acute and chronic change in [HCO_3^-]. In contrast to the acute (*chemical*) change, which would occur if we placed a beaker of blood into a gas-filled chamber with a low PCO_2, the chronic change is larger, more important, and *physiological* in nature. It arises from the compensatory activity of the kidney, which reduces [HCO_3^-] through a temporary decrease in bicarbonate regeneration and reabsorption. Both acute and chronic changes follow the same-direction rule.

Defects in Compensation: Terminology

Until now, I've assumed that if enough time elapses, compensation will always be present. But for compensation to develop, the physiological system (kidney or lung) that brings about the secondary change must be working properly. This is not always the case, especially in patients with complicated medical problems. When compensation is defective—partly or wholly absent—you can refer to the situation in several different ways. For example, consider a patient with metabolic acidosis whose respiratory compensation is impaired. You can refer to this situation using any of the following phrases: (1) metabolic acidosis with *inadequate compensation*, (2) metabolic acidosis with a *superimposed* respiratory acidosis (since PCO_2 is higher than it would be normally, it is correct to think of this as a respiratory acidosis), or (3) a *mixed* metabolic acidosis and respiratory acidosis. A similar variety of phrases can be used when speaking about defective compensation for the other primary disturbances. We'll focus on mixed disturbances in greater detail both later in this chapter and later in the book (especially in Chapters 10–13). Here I simply wanted to introduce a few terms and concepts, to smooth the way for what comes later.

Rules of thumb

To stabilize pH as effectively as possible, the body matches the intensity of the compensatory response to the severity of the underlying acid-base disorder. In fact, if you know the severity of the primary acid-base disorder, you can usually predict what the level of the compensatory variable will be. The easiest way to do this is with simple mathematical formulas, usually called **rules of thumb**. These rules summarize information obtained from research studies of normal compensation. The rules are useful clinically because if a patient has an acid-base disturbance, and you find that compensation is not at least roughly consistent with the level predicted by the rule, there is a good chance the disturbance is mixed. *The rules of thumb can thus tip you off to the presence of a mixed disturbance you otherwise might miss.*

In a moment, we'll study the rules in detail, but a few introductory comments will help make things clearer. If a patient's compensation is not as predicted, the situation necessarily takes one of two general forms: either the patient is **under-compensated** relative to the rule (that is, the compensatory variable has moved *too little* from its baseline; put differently, the compensated variable has remained too close to its starting level) or the patient is **overcompensated** relative to the rule (that is, the compensatory variable has moved *too much* from its baseline; put differently, compensation has overshot the predicted level). Let's look at what causes these two situations.

Undercompensation. If the patient is undercompensated, there are two possible explanations. Either (a) an additional disturbance is present—by definition, a mixed disturbance—or (b) more time is needed for compensation to develop fully. An example will clarify these two possibilities. Let's say a patient has metabolic acidosis and the rule of thumb tells you PCO_2 should be 25 mm Hg, but the actual PCO_2 is 34. Here, PCO_2 is decreased from normal, as predicted by the same-direction rule, but it is not low enough to satisfy the rule of thumb. One possibility (a) is that there is a superimposed respiratory acidosis (which tends to raise PCO_2). This respiratory acidosis is keeping PCO_2 from falling as far as it would otherwise.* This is a mixed disturbance: a combined metabolic acidosis and respiratory acidosis. The other possibility (b) is that more time is needed for PCO_2 to fall to its appropriate level. If this second possibility is at play, you'd expect that PCO_2 will continue to decline gradually till it reaches the predicted level. Based on the overall clinical situation, you'll need to figure out which of these two explanations (a or b) is most likely.

Overcompensation. If the patient is overcompensated, there is only one possible explanation: a mixed disturbance exists. Let's again say a patient has metabolic acidosis and the rule of thumb tells you PCO_2 should be 25, but this time the actual PCO_2 is 18. Once again, PCO_2 is decreased, as predicted by the same-direction rule, but this time it is too low: compensation has overshot the predicted level. The only possible explanation is a superimposed respiratory *alkalosis* (which is lowering PCO_2). Here, the mixed disturbance is a metabolic acidosis and a respiratory alkalosis. All this will become even clearer as you keep reading.

Let's now look at rules of thumb for the four primary disturbances. A variety of rules have been devised for each primary disturbance, all of which generate approximately the same predicted values. We'll focus on one popular rule for each of the primary disturbances. In studying this material, you'll be working through a lot of numerical information. If you're a first-time student of acid-base, don't try to retain everything right now. Instead, simply read for meaning—so that the concepts make sense as you encounter them—and do the calculations as you proceed. This will give you a solid foundation. Then, when we revisit the rules of thumb in Chapter 11 while learning blood gas interpretation formally, everything should fall smoothly into place.

---

* **Hint.** You can think of this situation additively: compensation lowers PCO_2 and the respiratory acidosis raises it. In this example, I assumed that the PCO_2-lowering effect of compensation is greater than the PCO_2-raising effect of the respiratory acidosis, which I'm assuming is relatively mild. Thus, the end, or net, result is that PCO_2 has decreased somewhat but not as far as predicted by the rule of thumb. Had the respiratory acidosis been more severe, it could have raised PCO_2 into the normal or even supranormal (hypercapnic) range.

Metabolic Acidosis

Rules of thumb for metabolic acidosis let you predict how low arterial PCO_2 should fall for a given primary decrease in arterial $[HCO_3^-]$. One well-known rule is referred to as the **Winters' formula**, after one of the researchers who developed it. The formula is:

$$\text{Compensated } PCO_2 = (1.5 \times \text{arterial } [HCO_3^-]) + 8$$

Here's an example. If metabolic acidosis reduces arterial $[HCO_3^-]$ to 16, you'd expect compensated arterial PCO_2 to be:

$$PCO_2 = (1.5 \times \text{arterial } [HCO_3^-]) + 8$$
$$PCO_2 = (1.5 \times 16) + 8$$
$$PCO_2 = 24 + 8$$
$$PCO_2 = 32$$

Because of patient-to-patient variability, the Winters' formula usually incorporates a plus/minus of 2, like this:

$$\text{Compensated } PCO_2 = (1.5 \times \text{arterial } [HCO_3^-]) + 8, \pm 2 \text{ mm Hg}$$

So, in the example just given, you'd expect a PCO_2 between 30 mm Hg (32 − 2 = 30) and 34 mm Hg (32 + 2 = 34). If PCO_2 were *not* in the 30–34 range, you'd suspect that a mixed disturbance was present. Specifically, you'd suspect that, in addition to the metabolic acidosis, there was a respiratory disturbance that caused PCO_2 to deviate from its expected level. A PCO_2 higher than expected (undercompensation) would—assuming enough time had passed for compensation to fully develop—point to respiratory acidosis. A PCO_2 lower than expected (overcompensation) would point to respiratory alkalosis.

For practice, look back to the profile for metabolic acidosis on page 57. Working with the numerical values given in that figure, determine whether the compensated PCO_2 lies within the range predicted by the Winters' formula. You can check your conclusion here.*

Metabolic Alkalosis

Rules of thumb for metabolic alkalosis let you predict how high arterial PCO_2 should rise for a given primary increase in arterial $[HCO_3^-]$. One well-known rule makes use of the number 0.7 and therefore can be thought of as **the 0.7 Rule**. The rule is:

$$PCO_2 \text{ rises } 0.7 \text{ mm Hg for each 1 mmol/l elevation in } [HCO_3^-]$$

---

*Answer—Metabolic Acidosis Profile.** The observed PCO_2 is 30, well within the 27–31 range predicted by the Winters' formula. Here's the Winters' calculation: $1.5 \times 14 = 21$. $21 + 8 = 29$. Building in the plus/minus range: $29 − 2 = 27$. $29 + 2 = 31$.

For example, if metabolic alkalosis increases $[HCO_3^-]$ by 10 mmol/l, you'd expect arterial PCO_2 to increase by about 7 mm Hg (10 x 0.7 = 7), to roughly 47, assuming a starting PCO_2 of 40. If $[HCO_3^-]$ increases by 15 mmol/l, you'd expect PCO_2 to be around 50 or 51. Compensation for metabolic alkalosis is highly variable, so a wide plus/minus range (usually ± 5) is generally built in. Therefore, you can give the formula like this:

PCO_2 rises 0.7 mm Hg for each 1 mmol/l elevation in $[HCO_3^-]$, ± 5 mm Hg

For example, if $[HCO_3^-]$ rises by 20 mmol/l from its normal level, PCO_2 should increase by about:

(20 x 0.7) ± 5
14 ± 5
14 − 5 = 9, 14 + 5 = 19
9 − 19

Therefore, the predicted compensated PCO_2 = 49–59, assuming a starting PCO_2 of 40.

For practice, look back to the profile for metabolic alkalosis on page 58. Does PCO_2 fall into the predicted range? Since you don't know the actual baseline values for this patient (this will be the case for many patients), use the midpoints of the normal ranges: baseline $[HCO_3^-]$ = 24, baseline PCO_2 = 40. Check your answer here.*

Respiratory Acidosis

Rules of thumb for respiratory acidosis let you predict how high compensatory $[HCO_3^-]$ should rise for a given primary increase in arterial PCO_2. Since there are both acute (chemical buffering) and chronic (renal compensation) changes in $[HCO_3^-]$, two rules are needed. For **acute** respiratory acidosis:

Each 10 mm Hg increase in PCO_2 causes $[HCO_3^-]$ to rise by 1 mmol/l

For example, if PCO_2 increases by 25 mm Hg (say, to 65 from an assumed baseline of 40), you'd expect $[HCO_3^-]$ to increase acutely by about 2.5 mmol/l—to about 26, from an assumed baseline of 24. For **chronic** respiratory acidosis:

Each 10 mm Hg elevation in PCO_2 raises $[HCO_3^-]$
between 3.5 mmol/l and 5.0 mmol/l

---

*Answer—Metabolic Alkalosis Profile. PCO_2 is within the predicted range of 43–53, calculated as follows. Assuming that the baseline $[HCO_3^-]$ is 24, you know that $[HCO_3^-]$ rose by 11 (35 − 24 = 11). Multiply 11 x 0.7 = 7.7, which rounds to 8. Adding 8 to the assumed baseline PCO_2 of 40 gives 48 (40 + 8 = 48). Build in the plus/minus: 48 − 5 = 43, 48 + 5 = 53. Had PCO_2 been above 53 (overcompensation), you'd suspect a superimposed respiratory acidosis. Had PCO_2 been below 43 (undercompensation), and enough time had passed for compensation to develop, you'd suspect a superimposed respiratory alkalosis.

This 3.5–5.0 range incorporates both the acute (chemical) change and the slower (physiological) change—so this rule lets you calculate the final expected $[HCO_3^-]$ in a patient with chronic respiratory acidosis. For example, if a COPD patient with chronic respiratory acidosis had a PCO_2 of 50 (10 mm Hg above an assumed baseline of 40), you'd expect the fully compensated arterial $[HCO_3^-]$ to be 3.5–5.0 mmol/l above its normal baseline set point. Assuming a baseline $[HCO_3^-]$ of 24 mmol/l, the compensated $[HCO_3^-]$ should be between 27.5 and 29 mmol/l. As with the other rules of thumb, these acute and chronic rules are only approximate, so you should allow $[HCO_3^-]$ to be slightly higher or lower than the expected range before assuming that a superimposed metabolic disturbance is present. (Most clinicians don't use explicit ranges, or plus/minus values, for the acute rule. They just calculate the predicted value and allow a bit of deviation in either direction.)

For practice, look back to the profile for respiratory acidosis on page 58. Are both acute and chronic PCO_2 as predicted?*

Respiratory Alkalosis

Rules for respiratory alkalosis let you predict how far compensatory $[HCO_3^-]$ will fall for a given primary decrease in arterial PCO_2. Again, there are separate rules for acute and chronic. For **acute** respiratory alkalosis:

> Each 10 mm Hg decline in PCO_2 reduces $[HCO_3^-]$ by 2 mmol/l

So, if PCO_2 falls by 15 mm Hg, you'd expect $[HCO_3^-]$ to fall by about 3 mmol/l. For **chronic** respiratory alkalosis:

> Each 10 mm Hg decline in PCO_2 reduces $[HCO_3^-]$ by 4 mmol/l

This 4 value incorporates both the acute (chemical) change and the slower (physiological) change. So, if a patient had chronic respiratory alkalosis with a PCO_2 of 30 mm Hg, you'd expect the final compensated arterial $[HCO_3^-]$ to be about 4 mmol/l below its normal set point (around 20 mmol/l, assuming a baseline of 24).

Once again, these rules are only approximate, so you should allow the observed values to be a bit higher or lower than predicted by the rule before assuming a

---

*Answer—respiratory acidosis profiles.** Both acute and chronic profiles are as predicted, as follows. *Acute.* Assuming a baseline PCO_2 of 40, PCO_2 rose acutely by 20 mm Hg. Since a 10 mm Hg increase in PCO_2 raises $[HCO_3^-]$ by 1 mmol/l, a 20 mm Hg increase raises $[HCO_3^-]$ by 2, from 24 to 26. The acute picture fits together. *Chronic:* A 20 mm Hg rise in PCO_2 should increase $[HCO_3^-]$ by 7–10 mm Hg, according to the rule. Assuming a starting $[HCO_3^-]$ of 24, the predicted $[HCO_3^-]$ is between 31 (24 + 7) and 34 (24 + 10). The observed value of 30 mmol/l is a bit low, but keep in mind that the baseline $[HCO_3^-]$ might actually have been as low as 21 since the normal arterial $[HCO_3^-]$ range is about 21–27 (p. 23). Had baseline $[HCO_3^-]$ been 21, the predicted compensatory range would be between 28 (21 + 7) and 31 (21 + 10). Since you won't always know the actual baseline values, there may be an element of clinically informed guesswork involved in situations like this.

mixed disturbance. For practice, look back to the profile for respiratory alkalosis on page 59. Are both acute and chronic PCO_2 as predicted?*

I'll say more about these rules—and you'll work additional practice problems using them—when we discuss blood gas interpretation in Chapter 11.

The rules of thumb just discussed are compiled in a table on page 130.

Summary

Compensation helps stabilize pH through a same-direction change in the "other" variable (i.e., PCO_2 or $[HCO_3^-]$). For example, metabolic acidosis, a primary fall in $[HCO_3^-]$, is compensated by a secondary fall in PCO_2. This secondary change returns the $[HCO_3^-]$-to-PCO_2 ratio, and hence pH, towards its normal value. During metabolic acid-base disturbances, ventilation begins to change within 30 minutes, and PCO_2 usually achieves its final compensated level within 12–24 hours. In contrast, the compensation for respiratory disturbances can take 3–5 days to complete. Compensation for metabolic disturbances, which affects PCO_2, is termed respiratory compensation, since the compensatory process is carried out by the respiratory system. Compensation for respiratory disturbances can be called either renal compensation (since it is carried out by the kidney) or metabolic compensation (since it affects bicarbonate level). Because compensation for respiratory disturbances develops slowly, it is important to distinguish between acute (uncompensated) and chronic (compensated) disturbances. Compensation is more complete for respiratory disturbances than for metabolic disturbances. That is, the $[HCO_3^-]$-to-PCO_2 ratio, and hence pH, is closer to normal. In respiratory disturbances (both acidosis and alkalosis), compensation can move pH into the normal range, though still not to its original baseline set point. In contrast, in metabolic disturbances, compensation cannot move pH into the normal range. The appropriate level of compensation can be predicted—at least roughly—using rules of thumb. These rules are summarized in the table on p. 130. Abnormal compensation takes one of two forms: undercompensation (the compensatory variable moved less from its baseline than expected) or overcompensation (the compensatory variable moved more from its baseline than expected). If undercompensation is present, there are two possible explanations: either a mixed disturbance exists or not enough time has elapsed for full compensation to develop. In contrast, if significant overcompensation is present, a mixed disturbance is the only possibility.

---

*__Answer—Respiratory Alkalosis Profiles.__ The acute profile is as expected. The chronic $[HCO_3^-]$ is a bit lower than you'd expect, but since it is still within a couple of mmol/l of the predicted value, you can probably attribute it to normal variation. In fact, this lowish $[HCO_3^-]$ is what brought pH into the normal range. But if $[HCO_3^-]$ had been much lower, you'd seriously consider the possibility of a superimposed metabolic acidosis.

Chapter 6

Metabolic Acidosis

In this chapter, we'll study metabolic acidosis in detail, focusing on its pathophysiology and on the clinical conditions that bring metabolic acidosis about. Towards the end of the chapter, we'll also discuss some laboratory tests and treatment concepts relevant to metabolic acidosis. As a reminder, metabolic acidosis is a disease process that decreases the bicarbonate concentration ($[HCO_3^-]$) of blood plasma, thereby producing acidemia. Any marked decline in plasma $[HCO_3^-]$—aside from that caused by the compensation for respiratory alkalosis—is by definition metabolic acidosis.*

The consequences of metabolic acidosis are not entirely clear. Although the evidence is not definitive, *acute* metabolic acidosis with a pH below 7.1 may impair cardiac contractility and cause arterial vasodilation, leading to hypotension. Acute metabolic acidosis with these low pH levels may also cause constriction of large veins, displacing blood into the pulmonary circulation, thereby raising pulmonary blood volume and pressure. These pulmonary hemodynamic changes—especially when occurring together with impaired cardiac contractility—might predispose the patient to congestive heart failure with pulmonary edema. The low pH may also increase susceptibility to serious ventricular arrhythmias. *Chronic* metabolic acidosis has different consequences, which we'll consider when discussing treatment concepts at the end of the chapter.

With that background, let's now dive in to the main part of the chapter, on the clinical causes and pathophysiology of metabolic acidosis. The clinical causes can be divided into four main categories:

1. Diarrhea
2. Organic acidoses (lactic acidosis, ketoacidosis)
3. Toxic ingestions (especially methanol, ethylene glycol, and salicylates)
4. Renal impairments (renal failure, renal tubular acidosis)

Let's consider these four categories individually.

Diarrhea

Take a moment to study the following figure, then refer back to it as you continue to read:

---

* **Terminology.** The term metabolic acidosis is introduced and fully explained in Chapter 2. For a quick refresher of the main point, see the illustration on page 28. The concept of compensation is explained in Chapter 5.

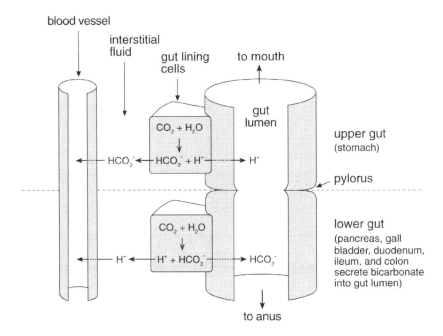

Notice that inside the cells which line the gut lumen, protons and bicarbonate are produced by the reaction $CO_2 + H_2O \rightarrow HCO_3^- + H^+$. (This same reaction occurs in the kidney, inside renal tubular cells, as we saw in Chapter 4.) In the stomach—that is, above the pylorus, indicated by the dashed line—the newly produced H^+ are secreted into the gut lumen, lowering the pH of stomach contents, and the newly produced HCO_3^- is secreted towards the blood and enters the ECF. In contrast, in most gut segments below the pylorus, the opposite ion movements occur: HCO_3^- is secreted into the gut lumen and H^+ is secreted towards the blood. This means that the lower gut adds protons to the ECF. These protons are buffered in the ECF by bicarbonate ($HCO_3^- + H^+ \rightarrow CO_2 + H_2O$). As a result, the functioning of the lower gut results in a gradual loss of bicarbonate from the ECF. (The CO_2 that is generated from the buffering reaction is eliminated at the lung during normal ventilation, so arterial PCO_2 does not rise.)

During normal digestion (i.e., no diarrhea), the ECF bicarbonate that gets lost due to the lower gut is replaced by two processes. First, as just described, cells lining the stomach add bicarbonate to blood. This stomach-produced bicarbonate makes up for most of the bicarbonate lost by the lower gut. Second, the remaining difference in bicarbonate is made up for by the kidney, as part of its normal bicarbonate regenerating activity (Chapter 4). Therefore, during normal gut function, plasma $[HCO_3^-]$ does not fall, even though the lower gut, viewed in isolation, does tend to acidify the body fluids.

However, during diarrhea, secretion by the lower gut increases, resulting in the loss of additional bicarbonate from the ECF. The increase in lower gut secretion is largely due to the greater volume of stool or diarrhea fluid. In addition, in some types of diarrhea (e.g. cholera) the infection or toxin directly stimulates the secretion of bicarbonate and other ions into the gut lumen. These additional losses of bicarbonate occur without a matching increase in secretion by the stomach, so plasma [HCO_3^-] tends to fall, resulting in metabolic acidosis. When diarrhea is severe, plasma [HCO_3^-] can fall to below 10 mmol/l.*

Potassium and other electrolytes. During diarrhea, loss of water and Na^+ in diarrhea fluid lowers ECF volume. This volume depletion, which can be severe, is sensed by the kidney, which responds by secreting renin. Renin secretion is the first step in the activation of the renin-angiotensin-aldosterone system, the final step of which is the secretion of aldosterone by the adrenal cortex. The resulting rise in plasma [aldosterone] feeds back on the kidney, stimulating it to increase sodium reabsorption. Increased sodium reabsorption is beneficial, in that it minimizes volume losses in the urine, which would otherwise exacerbate the volume depletion. However, the high plasma [aldosterone] also stimulates K^+ *secretion* by the renal tubule, leading to urinary K^+ losses. In addition, the high [aldosterone] also acts on the colon, causing it to secrete K^+ into the colonic lumen, and this K^+ is lost in the diarrhea fluid. As a result of these aldosterone-mediated effects on both the kidney and the colon, metabolic acidosis from diarrhea usually presents with *hypokalemia* (low plasma [K^+]).

It is important to understand that most potassium in the body is located inside cells: the [K^+] of intracellular fluid (ICF) is about 150 mmol/l, compared to a [K^+] in the ECF of roughly 4–5 mmol/l. During metabolic acidosis, as extracellular [HCO_3^-] falls, some intracellular HCO_3^- moves out of cells down its concentration gradient. As this HCO_3^- exits cells, it electrically attracts intracellular K^+ and drags it along into the ECF, thus maintaining electroneutrality (i.e., an equality of positive and negative charges) in both the ICF and ECF. Once this K^+ enters the ECF, it is susceptible to being eliminated in urine and stool. Because K^+ from both the ECF and ICF are lost in diarrhea, whole-body (ECF + ICF) K^+ losses can be substantial.**

Organic Acidoses (Lactic Acidosis and Ketoacidosis)

As part of normal metabolism, the body produces large quantities of organic acids. For example, lactic acid is produced at a rate of over 1000 mmols per day, mostly by the muscles. These organic acids are relatively strong (low pK) and thus dissociate almost completely, releasing protons and organic anions (e.g., lactate). The protons are buffered by bicarbonate ($HCO_3^- + H^+ \rightarrow CO_2 + H_2O$), with the CO_2 that is generated being eliminated at the lung. However—and this is a key point— plasma [HCO_3^-] does *not* fall. The reason is that the organic anions are carried by blood to the liver, where they are further metabolized to either glucose or to carbon dioxide and water. This additional metabolic step produces bicarbonate as a byproduct. In this step, the anion "disappears" and bicarbonate "appears," so—in terms of the net reaction—it looks as if the anion is transformed into bicarbonate

---

*Hint. Notice that during diarrhea, bicarbonate is not directly transferred from blood to intestinal lumen. However, the net result is the same: a loss of bicarbonate from blood, which lowers plasma [HCO_3^-], and a gain of bicarbonate in the intestinal lumen. As a mental shorthand, some people find it useful to think of diarrhea as involving a direct transfer of bicarbonate from blood to gut lumen.

** Clinical note. This explains why merely replacing the estimated extracellular losses (calculated as ECF Volume × Decrease in Plasma [K^+]) may not be adequate to replace all the lost potassium.

(Organic anion $\rightarrow$ HCO_3^-). Thus, as a short-hand, it is often said that organic anions are **"metabolized to bicarbonate."** This newly produced bicarbonate fully replaces the bicarbonate that was just lost during buffering.*

In certain disease states, however, an imbalance can develop in which organic acid production outpaces organic anion metabolism. This imbalance has three consequences. First, bicarbonate lost during buffering is not adequately replaced, so plasma $[HCO_3^-]$ falls. That is, metabolic acidosis develops. Second, the plasma concentration of the organic anion rises. Third, the rise in the plasma organic anions can lead to spillage of the anion in the urine. Such spillage occurs if the quantity of the anions filtered at the glomerulus exceeds the capacity of the renal tubule to reabsorb them. This spillage has important consequences: as long as the anions remain in the body, they can potentially be metabolized to bicarbonate at a later time, increasing $[HCO_3^-]$, but once the anions are excreted in the urine, the "potential bicarbonate" they represent is lost and must be replaced by other means (either by renal bicarbonate regeneration or by the clinician).

There are two common clinical settings in which organic acid production outpaces organic anion metabolism, resulting in metabolic acidosis: **lactic acidosis** and **ketoacidosis**. These conditions can be referred to generically as **organic acidoses** because they are caused by organic acids. Let's consider lactic acidosis and ketoacidosis individually.

Lactic Acidosis

Lactic acidosis is defined as metabolic acidosis caused by an imbalance between lactic acid production and lactate metabolism. Let's dissect this definition. **Lactic acid** is a 3-carbon organic acid that dissociates strongly in the body fluids, resulting in the organic anion, known as **lactate**, and a free proton. You can represent the dissociation like this: Lactic acid $\rightarrow$ Lactate$^-$ + H$^+$. Here are the structures of both lactic acid and lactate, in case you want to put a chemical "face" to the names:

$$ CH_3 - \overset{\overset{\text{OH}}{|}}{\underset{\underset{\text{H}}{|}}{C}} - COOH \longrightarrow CH_3 - \overset{\overset{\text{OH}}{|}}{\underset{\underset{\text{H}}{|}}{C}} - COO^- + H^+ $$

Lactic Acid   Lactate

---

*__Clinical note.__ The metabolism of organic anions to bicarbonate explains why lactate (the dissociated form of lactic acid) is included in Ringers lactate (a.k.a., Ringers solution or lactated Ringers), an intravenous fluid widely used in the surgical setting. In the body, so long as the normal metabolic pathways are active, the lactate in Ringer's solution is metabolized to bicarbonate and thus has the same acid-base effect as giving bicarbonate itself. Lactate is used instead of bicarbonate because Ringers solution also contains calcium ions (Ca^{2+}), which can precipitate (i.e., form a non-dissolved solid) when bicarbonate is present. Understanding these issues also helps explain why vegetarian diets are usually associated with slightly higher plasma $[HCO_3^-]$ levels than meat-containing diets: not only do vegetarian diets contain lower levels of sulfur-containing amino acids, which are metabolized to sulfuric acid and thus consume bicarbonate, but fruits and vegetables contain high levels of organic anions, such as citrate, which are metabolized to bicarbonate after being absorbed by the gut.

Lactic acid is produced by the tissues during anaerobic metabolism (metabolism carried out in the absence of oxygen). Thus, lactic acid is rapidly produced during tissue hypoxia (low tissue PO_2), which most commonly results from either hypoxemia (low blood oxygen levels) or ischemia (inadequate blood flow to tissues). Adequate oxygen and blood flow are also necessary for the hepatic metabolism of lactate, because lactate metabolism is an oxidative process, and because normal blood flow is required to carry lactate to the liver in the first place. Thus, a general decrease in either tissue perfusion (blood flow) or oxygenation causes *both* an increase in lactic acid production *and* a decrease in lactate consumption. The result is a fall in plasma $[HCO_3^-]$—metabolic acidosis—and a rise in plasma [lactate].

The most common clinical cause of lactic acidosis is **septic shock** from systemic infection, which impairs tissue perfusion and thus reduces oxygen delivery to tissues. Some less common conditions that cause lactic acidosis are summarized in the following table. Reading through the table, you'll see that in many cases the bottom line is that the tissues are not getting enough oxygen.

Less Common Causes of Lactic Acidosis*	
Condition	**Pathophysiologic Mechanisms**
Severe acute hypoxemia	Leads to anaerobic metabolism and inability to metabolize lactate. Chronic hypoxemia usually does not cause lactic acidosis because increased hematocrit and chemical changes in blood (increased [2,3 DPG]) lead to more efficient oxygen delivery.
Severe convulsions	Increased muscle activity accompanied by hypoxemia from respiratory arrest (standstill).
Strenuous exercise, especially with dehydration	Increased lactic acid production from anaerobic metabolism. Volume depletion from dehydration hinders blood flow to both muscles (causing tissue hypoxia) and liver (causing tissue hypoxia and impairing lactate delivery).
Carbon monoxide (CO) poisoning	CO occupies oxygen-carrying sites on hemoglobin, reducing oxygen delivery to tissues.
Severe anemia	Reduces oxygen-carrying capacity. Iron-deficiency anemia also inhibits iron-dependent steps in the cellular use of oxygen.
Malignancies	Especially some leukemias, lymphomas, and small cell lung cancer. Metabolically active tumors can outstrip blood supply and oxygen delivery, leading to anaerobic metabolism. If tumor is present in the liver, metabolism of lactate may be impaired.
Diabetes Mellitus	Most commonly causes ketoacidosis but occasionally also causes lactic acidosis, partly because uncontrolled diabetes can lead to severe volume depletion, which can impair tissue perfusion.

table continued on next page

Severe liver disease such as cirrhosis	Impaired lactate metabolism.
Drugs	Various drugs can cause lactic acidosis as a specific adverse reaction. Two common examples are isoniazid and anti-retroviral drugs. In addition, any drug overdose that causes either cardiovascular collapse (low perfusion) or severe suppression of ventilation (hypoxemia) can cause lactic acidosis.
Severe heart failure	Reduced circulation and tissue perfusion results in decreased oxygen delivery.
Hemorrhagic shock	Reduced circulation and tissue perfusion results in decreased oxygen delivery.
Cardiogenic shock	Used to be common following myocardial infarction (MI); much less common now that acute MI is treated by immediate interventions such as balloon angioplasty.
* The most common cause of lactic acidosis is septic shock from systemic infection.	

In discussions of lactic acidosis, you may encounter the terms **Type A** and **Type B**. Type A lactic acidosis refers to those causes that involve obvious impairments of tissue perfusion or oxygenation. Type B lactic acidosis refers to all other causes. The division between Type A and B is imperfect, in that subtle hypoperfusion is present in some seemingly Type B causes. But the distinction between Type A and B is still sometimes used.

Potassium status in lactic acidosis. Uncomplicated lactic acidosis usually presents with a relatively normal $[K^+]$. However, complicating factors may cause plasma $[K^+]$ to rise, in particular during shock. Shock can impair renal perfusion, reducing renal K^+ excretion. Simultaneously, shock can cause tissue ischemia, injuring cells and leading them to release K^+ into the ECF.

Ketoacidosis

Let's start with some terminology. The term **ketoacid** refers to two related 4-carbon organic acids: **acetoacetic acid** and **beta-hydroxybutyric acid**. Only the first of these actually has a keto group in its chemical structure, but the name ketoacid is still used for both. Here are the structures:

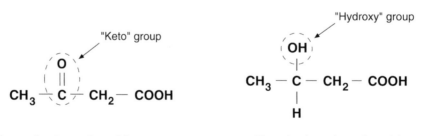

Acetoacetic acid   Beta-hydroxybutyric acid

Both acids dissociate almost completely in the ECF, leading to buffering by bicarbonate. (As with all organic acids, the H^+ comes from the COOH group.) This dissociation leaves behind **acetoacetate** and **beta-hydroxybutyrate**, the so-called **ketoacid anions**. Another substance, **acetone**, which is not an acid, is produced along with the two ketoacids. Acetone looks like this:

$$CH_3 - \overset{\overset{\textstyle O}{\|}}{C} - CH_3$$

Acetone

Ketone body is the general name given to acetone and the two ketoacids or their dissociated anions.

Ketoacidosis refers to the metabolic acidosis caused by an overproduction of ketoacids. It presents with low plasma $[HCO_3^-]$ and high plasma and urine levels of ketoacid anions. Ketoacidosis arises due to an abnormal hormonal milieu consisting of low plasma levels of insulin and high plasma levels of glucagon. Low insulin causes fat cells to release fatty acids into the blood, which flood the liver. High glucagon causes liver cells to metabolize these fatty acids via a ketogenic (ketone-producing) biochemical pathway. Glucagon is sometimes referred to as a "counter-regulatory hormone" because it opposes the action of insulin. Other counter-regulatory hormones also exist (e.g., epinephrine, cortisol) and high levels of these can sometimes contribute to ketoacidosis as well. Three main clinical situations are associated with low insulin and high glucagon and thus can result in ketoacidosis. These are:

Diabetic Ketoacidosis (DKA). If an insulin-dependent diabetic (type 1 diabetes) does not receive adequate insulin, severe ketoacidosis with very low plasma $[HCO_3^-]$ can result. Plasma [glucose] is usually very high, leading to spillage of glucose in the urine.

Starvation Ketoacidosis. Starvation suppresses insulin and raises glucagon secretion, and can therefore cause ketoacidosis. This ketoacidosis develops gradually: it is usually apparent after several days without food but may not peak for two weeks. Even at its peak, the acidosis is usually mild ($[HCO_3^-]$ rarely drops below about 18 mmol/l) and does not generally require specific therapy. Starvation ketoacidosis can also arise from deliberate fasting or anorexia nervosa.

Alcoholic Ketoacidosis (AKA). With a prolonged drinking-vomiting binge, decreased food intake and vomiting, which empties residual food from the stomach, effectively produces starvation ketoacidosis. Ketogenesis is intensified by (a) a high plasma level of catecholamines, which arises as a response to volume depletion from vomiting, and (b) a direct effect of alcohol. Plasma [glucose] may be low, normal, or moderately elevated. Plasma $[HCO_3^-]$ can be very low.

In all types of ketoacidosis, plasma levels of ketoacid anions rise, and large amounts of the anions spill into the urine. These anions, and the cations (especially Na^+) that are excreted with them to maintain electroneutrality, are all osmotically active,

73

so they drag water into the urine and sharply increase urine output ("osmotic diuresis"). In DKA, urinary glucose spillage has the same osmotic effect, further increasing fluid losses. As a result, polyuria (abnormally high urine output) is typical of DKA and frequently results in severe volume depletion, which in turn leads to polydipsia (abnormally increased thirst and fluid intake).

Potassium status in DKA. Potassium status in DKA is an important clinical topic, so I'm going to say a lot about it. In DKA, as in diarrhea, volume depletion activates the renin-angiotensin-aldosterone system (p. 69). As in diarrhea, the resulting rise in plasma [aldosterone] promotes urinary K^+ excretion. This urinary K^+ loss is exacerbated by the osmotic diuresis, which moves water rapidly through the nephron. Also as in diarrhea, much of the lost K^+ comes from inside cells.

In DKA, K^+ exits cells by three specific mechanisms. First, insulin is necessary to maintain normal intracellular $[K^+]$. (Insulin stimulates the Na^+–K^+–ATPase, which transports K^+ into cells.) Therefore, when insulin is low, cellular K^+ leaks into the ECF. Second, high plasma [glucose] raises plasma osmolarity, which draws water out of cells. As water exits cells, it carries K^+ with it by a process known as "solvent drag." Third, this osmotic loss of water from cells causes $[K^+]$ inside cells to increase. The increased intracellular $[K^+]$ promotes the exit of K^+ into the ECF through potassium channels in the cell membrane. By moving cellular K^+ into the ECF, these three mechanisms expose additional K^+ to urinary excretion.* Therefore, in DKA, total-body (ECF + ICF) K^+ losses are very large.

So far, the situation sounds much like diarrhea, which also involves substantial total-body losses of K^+, even if different mechanisms cause the K^+ to exit cells. However, in DKA, there is usually a paradoxical finding: although the patients are often badly K^+ depleted, hypokalemia occurs in only a small fraction of patients. The vast majority present with a plasma $[K^+]$ that is either *normal* or *elevated*. Often, plasma $[K^+]$ is in the range of 5–6 mmol/l. (Normal plasma $[K^+]$ is about 3.5–5.0 mmol/l.) The reason: at the same time K^+ is lost from the ECF via the urine, a large amount of K^+ enters the ECF from inside cells. The final plasma $[K^+]$ depends on how much K^+ is lost in urine *compared to* how much K^+ enters the ECF from inside cells. The relative rates of these two types of K^+ movements (cell-to-ECF, ECF-to-urine) vary, but in most patients the cell-to-ECF movements offset, or more than offset, the urinary losses, so hypokalemia does not occur.

This leads us to three important clinical points. First, in almost all DKA patients, regardless of the plasma $[K^+]$ level, total-body (ECF + ICF) K^+ stores are greatly reduced. Second, the administration of insulin reverses the mechanisms that caused K^+ to leave cells, so some K^+ shifts back into cells. Therefore, plasma $[K^+]$ can plummet acutely, since the $[K^+]$ level now suddenly reflects whole-body K^+

---

*__Going further.__ Notice that I did *not* refer to the mechanism I previously described for diarrhea: the exit of intracellular K^+ to maintain electroneutrality as bicarbonate moves out of cells. In the organic acidoses, the organic anions readily enter cells when HCO_3^- exits, thus balancing the charge without the need for K^+ to exit. In contrast, in diarrhea and other so-called *in*organic acidoses (e.g., renal failure, RTA), the excess anion is chloride, which does not readily enter cells. Thus, when bicarbonate exits cells, the negative charge must be balanced by the exit of intracellular K^+.

depletion. Thus, giving insulin, although necessary, can result in severe hypokalemia. Third, to prevent this acute hypokalemia from developing, DKA patients are usually given K^+ as part of the treatment protocol, thus repleting body K^+ stores even before plasma $[K^+]$ has a chance to fall.

In alcoholic ketoacidosis (AKA), plasma $[K^+]$ can be high, normal, or low. However, unlike in DKA, AKA patients do not usually have large whole-body K^+ deficits.

Toxic Ingestions (Salicylates, Methanol, and Ethylene Glycol)

Three widely available substances—salicylates, methanol, and ethylene glycol—can cause metabolic acidosis by unique mechanisms. We will consider these individually.

Salicylates: Aspirin and Related Substances

Overdose with salicylates can cause both metabolic acidosis and respiratory alkalosis (i.e., a mixed disturbance). The respiratory alkalosis often develops first and sometimes presents as a simple (not mixed) disturbance. Then the metabolic acidosis develops. In adults, two clinical pictures are common: (a) metabolic acidosis and respiratory alkalosis are of equal severities, resulting in a roughly normal plasma pH; and (b) the respiratory alkalosis predominates, resulting in a high plasma pH. In children, the respiratory alkalosis is often mild, so the metabolic acidosis typically predominates, resulting in a low plasma pH. Scan this figure, then refer back to it as you keep reading:

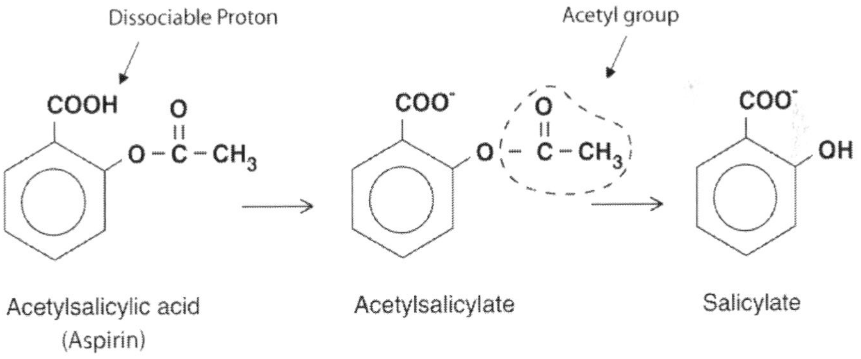

Salicylates are usually ingested as acetylsalicylic acid (ordinary aspirin, a.k.a. ASA—the structure on the left), which rapidly dissociates (loss of the acid proton) to acetylsalicylate (the middle structure). Notice that the acetyl group is then removed from the acetylsalicylate, converting it to salicylate (structure on right); this conversion takes place in the liver. It is the salicylate that causes the acid-base disturbances. Salicylate interferes with various enzymes, leading to increased production of organic acids, especially keto- and lactic acids. These acids are a major cause of the metabolic acidosis. Though protons released from the dissociation of acetylsalicylic acid are buffered by bicarbonate, the amount of aspirin typically ingested reduces $[HCO_3^-]$ only slightly by this route. Respiratory alkalosis occurs because salicylate directly stimulates the respiratory center in the medulla of the brain stem, causing hyperventilation. Many non-prescription products contain aspirin, including Alka-Seltzer, Maalox, and Pepto-Bismol. Topical pain relievers (e.g. oil of wintergreen, Bengay) and wart removers (salicylic acid) often contain large amounts of salicylate, and toxic doses of salicylate can be absorbed if these substances are applied to large areas of skin.

Methanol and Ethylene Glycol

Methanol (a.k.a. methyl alcohol, wood alcohol) is widely used as an industrial solvent and as an anti-freeze ingredient, including in car windshield washing solutions. Ethylene glycol, another industrial solvent, is an ingredient of car radiator antifreeze solutions. Because ethylene glycol is odorless and tastes sweet, children and pets sometimes drink it, and it is occasionally used illegally to sweeten wine. Methanol and ethylene glycol are not acids and neither is directly toxic. However, both are metabolized to toxic acids and other products that can cause severe acidosis and other lethal effects. As little as 50 ml (1 tablespoon = 15 ml) of either methanol or ethylene glycol can kill an adult, and as little as 10 ml can cause toxicity.

The following figure shows the metabolism of methanol and ethylene glycol to toxic products. Study this figure, and then refer back to it as you continue reading:

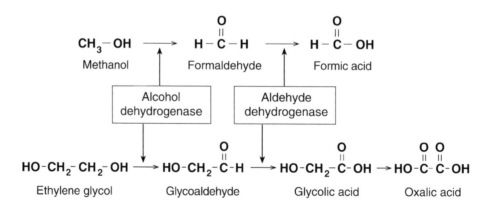

In this figure, the two boxes give the names of enzymes involved in the metabolism. As you can see, the same enzymes metabolize both methanol and ethylene glycol. This makes sense, since the chemical structures of methanol and ethylene glycol are somewhat similar; both have an alcohol (-OH) group attached to a carbon atom. Notice that the primary toxic end products are formic acid (for methanol) and glycolic acid and oxalic acid (for ethylene glycol). These toxic acids accumulate in the body fluids. They can cause metabolic acidosis directly when they dissociate. They also poison other metabolic pathways and lead to the production of lactic acid and other acids. The two enzymes boxed in the above figure are also the same enzymes that metabolize ordinary drinking alcohol (ethanol). For this reason, ethanol has traditionally been given as part of the immediate treatment for methanol and ethylene glycol ingestion. The ethanol competes with the methanol and ethylene glycol at the enzyme's active sites, keeping the enzyme occupied and thus slowing the conversion of methanol and ethylene glycol to toxic products. With this partial protection in place, the patient can be dialyzed to remove the remaining methanol and ethylene glycol from the body.*

Potassium status in methanol, ethylene glycol, and salicylate intoxication. With these three toxins, plasma [K^+] can be normal, high, or low. When hyperkalemia (high plasma [K^+]) or hypokalemia do occur, they tend to be relatively mild. However, ethylene glycol is metabolized to oxalate, which can bind with calcium ions, forming calcium oxalate crystals. These crystals deposit in many tissues in the body, including the kidneys, where they can cause acute renal failure. If renal failure occurs, hyperkalemia can be severe due to impaired urinary K^+ excretion.

Renal Impairments (Renal Failure, Renal Tubular Acidosis)

The kidney carries out two main processes involving bicarbonate: reabsorption and regeneration (discussed in detail in Chapter 4). If either process is impaired, metabolic acidosis results. If reabsorption fails, filtered bicarbonate spills into the urine, reducing plasma [HCO_3^-]. If regeneration fails, the kidney can't adequately replace bicarbonate that is lost while buffering the normal load of endogenously produced acid (p. 40), so [HCO_3^-] falls gradually. Both reabsorption and regeneration are carried out by the renal tubule, in particular by the renal tubular cells. There are two main conditions that impair the renal tubule's handling of bicarbonate and thus cause metabolic acidosis: **renal failure** and **renal tubular acidosis (RTA)**. Let's consider these individually.

Renal Failure

Renal failure, which can be either acute or chronic, has many different causes. The shared and defining feature is a marked reduction in glomerular filtration rate (GFR), which leads to a marked rise in plasma levels of nitrogenous (nitrogen containing) wastes such as creatinine and urea.** In chronic renal failure, creatinine levels of 10 mg/dl or higher are common (normal is about 1 mg/dl). Plasma levels of several non-nitrogenous anions—including sulfate, phosphate, and various organic anions—also frequently rise. Dialysis is often considered once creatinine reaches 5 or 6 mg/dl.

Renal failure is defined by the impairment in GFR and, strictly speaking, metabolic acidosis is not intrinsic to the definition. Still, metabolic acidosis develops as renal failure progresses. In many patients, metabolic acidosis is present by the time GFR falls to about 1/4th its normal level, which is reflected in a roughly 4-fold rise

---

*__Clinical note.__ It is now much more common to give the drug fomepizole, which has about the same effect as ethanol but without producing inebriation. It is still appropriate to give ethanol in settings when fomepizole is not available.

** **Terminology.** High plasma levels of nitrogenous (nitrogen-containing) waste is referred to as azotemia (from the French, *azote*, "nitrogen"). Creatinine and urea, which is usually measured as blood urea nitrogen (BUN), are the nitrogenous wastes most commonly measured. Therefore, BUN and creatinine serve as laboratory markers for azotemia.

in plasma creatinine from its baseline level. However, there is considerable variability from patient to patient, so you really can't predict at what point metabolic acidosis will develop.

How does renal failure cause metabolic acidosis? The primary mechanism is a *decrease in ammonium excretion* by the renal tubule. Ammonium excretion is the kidney's major route for regenerating bicarbonate. During severe renal failure, ammonium excretion falls to between 0.5 and 15 mmol per day. When you consider that these levels occur during metabolic acidosis—which normally stimulates a homeostatic increase in ammonium excretion to levels that can exceed 400 mmol/day—the extent of the decline becomes apparent. The decline in ammonium excretion occurs largely because of a reduction in the total number of functioning nephrons. This loss of nephrons is often referred to as "nephronal dropout." Because this dropout involves the entire nephron, it affects both glomerular filtration (resulting in a rise in BUN and creatinine) and tubular function (resulting in metabolic acidosis).

Potassium status in renal failure. The loss of functioning nephrons slows urinary K^+ excretion at least somewhat. Therefore, renal failure tends to raise plasma $[K^+]$. This elevation is usually mild, with $[K^+]$ often remaining in the normal range (high-normal). However, if a substantial amount of K^+ acutely enters the ECF, frank hyperkalemia can develop, which usually resolves gradually as the kidneys slowly excrete the excess K^+. Common causes of acute K^+ loads include intravenous potassium, tissue breakdown with release of intracellular K^+, and use of KCl-containing salt substitutes (e.g., "lite salt").

Renal Tubular Acidosis (RTA)

The name Renal Tubular Acidosis (RTA) conveys the essence of the disease: a *renal* disorder that affects the *tubules* and causes *metabolic acidosis.* As the adjective *tubular* implies, impairments in glomerular filtration are not central to the disease. Therefore, in sharp contrast to renal failure, GFR is either normal or reduced only modestly and, as a result, plasma [creatinine] is either normal or only modestly elevated. You can think of RTA as any renal acidosis that is not associated with a major impairment in GFR.

Renal tubular acidosis is not really a single disease. Rather, it is an umbrella term applied to perhaps a dozen different entities with distinct pathophysiologies, all of which are renal, tubular, and acidosis-causing. Because it is not easy to distinguish among some of these entities, it is usual to categorize RTA into three broad groups, called "types," and to limit the initial diagnosis to differentiating among the three. The types are numbered 1, 2, and 4. (For historical reasons, the term Type 3 is not used.) RTA is uncommon—much less common than renal failure—so I'll compress detailed information about the types into a table. Much of this table is included largely for reference. However, even as a first-time student of acid-base, you should study the first three rows (*Children vs. Adult, Plasma Creatinine,* and *Plasma [K+])*, as these are the differentiating features you're most likely to encounter clinically.

Renal Tubular Acidosis

	Type 1 (a.k.a. Distal RTA)	Type 2 (a.k.a. Proximal RTA)	Type 4 (a.k.a. Hyperkalemic RTA)
Children vs. Adult	Rare in both children and adults	Most common RTA in children	Most common RTA in adults
Plasma Creatinine	Normal	Normal	Moderately elevated. Often 1.5–2.0 mg/dl
Plasma [K+]	Usually low (but may be normal)	Usually low (but may be normal)	High
Plasma [HCO$_3^-$]	Often below 10 mmol/l	Typically 15–20 mmol/l	Typically 15–20 mmol/l
Pathophysiology	Defect in distal tubule impairs ability to reduce pH in distal luminal fluid. As a result, urine pH is relatively high. Plasma [K+] is low due to urinary spillage of K+.	Defect in proximal tubule impairs ability to reabsorb HCO$_3^-$ from proximal luminal fluid. HCO$_3^-$ spills in urine until plasma [HCO$_3^-$] falls to a level where all bicarbonate can again be reabsorbed. Plasma [K+] is low due to urinary spillage of K+.	Most often caused by low aldosterone secretion, often secondary to low renin secretion by the kidney ("hyporeninemic hypoaldosteronism"). Low [aldosterone] and low GFR both impair K+ excretion, raising plasma [K+].
Urine pH	Above 5.3	Two stages. Early on, while plasma [HCO$_3^-$] is falling to its new level due to urinary bicarbonate spillage, pH is above 5.5. Once plasma [HCO$_3^-$] stabilizes at its new level due to cessation of urinary bicarbonate spillage, pH is below 5.5.	Below 5.3
Causes (partial listing)	Causes include Sjögren's and other autoimmune diseases, rare genetic defects, sickle cell disease, drugs (e.g., lithium, amphotericin B, ifosfamide), and exposure to toluene. (Toluene is a solvent found in some paints, thinners, rubber cement, and airplane glue; toxicity can occur by ingestion, skin exposure, or deliberate sniffing.)	May occur alone or as part of generalized proximal reabsorptive dysfunction (Fanconi syndrome), which causes urinary spillage of many substances (HCO$_3^-$, phosphate, glucose, amino acids, uric acid, Na+, K+). Type 2 RTA can also be caused by drugs (e.g., acetazolamide, outdated tetracycline), toxins (lead, mercury, cadmium), and genetic abnormalities (e.g., Wilson's disease).	Usually caused by pathologies that interfere with the renin-angiotensin-aldosterone system, including: diabetic kidney disease (which impairs renin secretion), other renal causes (tubulo-interstitial kidney disease), and drugs (e.g., beta blockers, NSAIDs, COX-2 and ACE inhibitors).

Specific Diagnostic Tests

In this chapter and the next (on metabolic alkalosis), we'll briefly consider a number of *specific* laboratory tests that help you identify the *underlying cause* of the primary disturbance. The more *general* acid-base tests, such as the arterial blood gas and the anion gap—which are so important that they deserve full, step-by-step explanations—are presented in Chapters 11 and 12.

Diarrhea

Diarrhea is usually diagnosed by history or by physical exam evidence, such as soiled clothing or bedding, without the need for specific laboratory tests.

Lactic Acidosis

Lactic acidosis is diagnosed when the *plasma lactate level* is elevated, especially if the level approaches 5 mmol/liter. The normal range for plasma lactate is around 0.5–2.2 mmol/l. Urine lactate is typically normal because the kidney reabsorbs practically all lactate that is filtered, so virtually none spills into the urine.

Renal Failure

Renal failure is usually detected by a markedly elevated *creatinine and BUN*. Creatinine is often 10 mg/dl or higher (> 900 micromoles/liter). Normal ranges are creatinine 0.6–1.5 mg/dl and BUN 8–25 mg/dl.

Renal Tubular Acidosis (RTA)

RTA is usually first entertained as a diagnosis when you cannot attribute the metabolic acidosis to a more common cause. Once an RTA is suspected, the particular type can often be distinguished based on information given in the table on page 79.

Ketoacidosis

Ketones. Ketoacidosis usually gives a positive ketone test in both plasma and urine. Because ketones are more concentrated in urine than plasma, urine tests sometimes read positive even when plasma levels are quite low and therefore read negative, such as during mild starvation ketoacidosis. For this reason, it is often useful to confirm a positive urine ketone test with a plasma test. One limitation to most ketone tests is that they detect acetoacetate but not beta-hydroxybuyrate. This can be a problem in alcoholic ketoacidosis (AKA), and when ketoacidosis and lactic acidosis occur together ("keto-lactic acidosis"), because in these conditions much of the acetoacetate is converted to beta-hydroxybutyrate, so the test can give false negatives. In some hospitals, a plasma test for beta-hydroxybutyrate is available and can be used if you think the standard ketone test might be leading you astray.*

---

*Going further.** Most ketone assays—including plasma tests, urine dipsticks, and urine tests such as the Acetest (a brand name sometimes used loosely to refer to urine ketone

Glucose. In DKA, plasma glucose is typically 400 mg/dl (22 mmol/l) or higher but may occasionally be lower. Urine glucose is positive as well. A tentative diagnosis of DKA can be made at the bedside if a urine dipstick test is strongly positive for both ketones and glucose. In AKA, plasma glucose has no consistent level. It may be low, normal, or moderately elevated, occasionally reaching the low end of the range found in DKA (~400 mg/dl).

Acetone on the Breath. Acetone readily converts to a gas, so it is eliminated by the lung. Thus, the scent of acetone on the breath raises the possibility of ketoacidosis. Acetone smells a bit like nail polish remover, since it is the primary solvent in most brands, though added perfumes may obscure the true scent somewhat. Because plasma [acetone] is low even in severe ketoacidosis, the scent is not always detectable, so its absence does not rule out ketoacidosis.*

Methanol, Ethylene glycol, or Salicylate

If you suspect poisoning with methanol, ethylene glycol, or salicylate, order assays that are specific for the substance in question. Often you'll want to order all three assays, in addition to other standard toxicology screens. Finding any level of methanol or ethylene glycol suggests poisoning, but low levels of salicylate may be due to the therapeutic use of aspirin or other salicylates for pain relief. Most hospitals can test for salicylate. In contrast, many hospitals lack the specialized equipment (gas chromatography, GC) needed to test for methanol and ethylene glycol—and some hospitals that do have GC run the tests only once a day. When specific assays are not rapidly available (and sometimes even when they are), the following four procedures are useful: (1) calculate the osmolar gap, (2) check eyes, (3) examine urine for crystals, and (4) examine urine for fluorescence. We'll now look at each of these individually. A key point for these procedures is that while a positive test helps confirm the presence of a toxin, a negative test does *not* rule the toxin out.

Osmolar Gap

The plasma **osmolar gap** (a.k.a. osmo*lal* gap) helps you determine if an abnormal substance (e.g. methanol or ethylene glycol) is causing plasma osmolarity to be elevated. You can find the osmolar gap in three steps. First, using plasma values for Na^+, glucose, and BUN from an ordinary venous blood sample, find "calculated osmolarity" with this formula:

$$\text{Calculated osmolarity} = (2 \times [Na^+]) + ([glucose]/18) + (BUN/2.8)$$

---

assays in general)—quantify ketones using a substance called nitroprusside, which does not react with beta-hydroxybutyrate. In addition to lab-run tests for plasma beta-hydroxybutyrate, some sophisticated home testing devices for diabetics can now measure both glucose and beta-hydroxybutyrate in 30 seconds from a finger-stick capillary blood sample. These testers are available in some hospitals.

***Clinical note.** Acetone also is present in plasma, and can be detected on the breath, following ingestion of acetone or isopropyl alcohol, which is metabolized to acetone. However, acetone from these sources do not cause metabolic acidosis.

Calculated osmolarity quantifies that portion of total osmolarity that is due to substances that are *normally* present in blood.* Second, directly measure the *actual* osmolarity of blood plasma. This is done using a device called an osmometer, which most hospital labs have. This measured value is called "measured osmolarity." Third, to find the osmolar gap, subtract calculated osmolarity from measured osmolarity:

Osmolar gap = measured osmolarity – calculated osmolarity

The osmolar gap lets you compare predicted (calculated) osmolarity and actual (measured) osmolarity, with the objective of seeing if a toxic substance might be contributing to actual osmolarity. The normal range for the osmolar gap runs from -10 to +10 milliosmoles per liter (mOsm/l), a range of 20 mOsm/l. A gap above +10 mOsm/l level suggests that an abnormal uncharged (non-ionic) substance, such as methanol or ethylene glycol, is present in plasma. Methanol and ethylene glycol are so toxic, and the normal range of the osmolar gap is so wide, that low but lethal levels of these toxins can "hide" within the gap's normal range. Thus, while an elevated osmolar gap can suggest the presence of these toxins, a normal osmolar gap does <u>not</u> rule them out. When the time comes to actually use the osmolar gap clinically, it's helpful to know some additional fine points. These are contained in the box below. If you're a first-time student of acid-base, you might want to skip this box for now, to avoid getting bogged down in details.

The Osmolar Gap: Clinical Fine Points

1) All abnormal, uncharged (non-ionic) substances can elevate the osmolar gap. Only some of these substances cause metabolic acidosis. The following all raise the osmolar gap but don't cause metabolic acidosis: ethanol (drinking alcohol), isopropyl alcohol (rubbing alcohol), acetone (the non-ionic ketone body, which can be produced from either ketoacidosis or as the end product of isopropyl alcohol metabolism), and propylene glycol (a dilutant commonly used in the formulation of liquid medications, both p.o. and i.v.; the propylene glycol level is most likely to be elevated in ICU patients, who tend to receive many liquid medications). In addition, there is some evidence that patients with chronic renal failure who do not receive dialysis, as well as some patients with lactic acidosis, can have osmolar gaps up to about 20 mOsm/l. Hyperproteinemia and hyperlipidemia can also raise the osmolar gap. Thus, *the osmolar gap must be interpreted in light of the entire clinical picture.* Simply finding an elevated osmolar gap does not automatically indicate methanol or ethylene glycol.

---

*Going further. [Na^+] is doubled to take account of the plasma anions (largely chloride and bicarbonate) that balance the charges on sodium. Thus, doubling [Na^+] gives you a quick way to estimate the concentration, and hence the osmotic contribution, of all ions in the plasma. Since glucose and urea are the two main neutral (non-ionic) substances found in normal plasma, the formula incorporates the approximate osmotic contribution of normally present neutral substances as well. Using 18 and 2.8 as denominators converts these values from milligrams per deciliter (mg/dl), which is how they are reported by the lab in most U.S. hospitals, into mmol/l. This conversion is needed since it is the concentration of particles, which is what mmol/l measures, that determines osmolarity.

2) If you think a patient may have ingested *both* ethanol *and* a toxic substance such as methanol or ethylene glycol (a frequent combination), you can measure ethanol directly by the widely available enzymatic assay and then adjust the formula for calculated osmolarity to:

$$\text{Calculated osmolarity} = (2 \times [Na^+]) + ([glucose]/18) + (BUN/2.8) + (ethanol/4.6)$$

Using this formula, ethanol has no effect on the osmolar gap; that is, an elevation in the osmolar gap will indicate a substance *other* than ethanol.

3) The formulas given so far for calculated osmolarity assume you are measuring glucose, urea (BUN), and ethanol in mg/dl. If your lab reports these values in mmol/l, you should use the simpler formula:

$$\text{Calculated osmolarity} = (2 \times [Na^+]) + [glucose] + [urea] + [ethanol]$$

4) Some labs do a dangerous thing: if you request an osmolarity measurement, they *calculate* the osmolarity—using the same formula for calculated osmolarity given above—instead of measuring it. If you unwittingly use this calculated value as your measured value in determining the osmolar gap, you'll always get 0 (because you'll actually be subtracting calculated osmolarity from itself), no matter what toxins are present. Make sure the lab gives you a true *measured* osmolarity.

5) There are two kinds of osmometers: vapor pressure and freezing-point suppression. Vapor pressure osmometers can detect the osmotic contribution of ethylene glycol but not of methanol or other alcohols. Freezing-point suppression osmometers can detect all these substances. Know what kind of osmometer your lab has. Vapor pressure osmometers can lead to false negatives for toxic alcohols and should be replaced.

6) Ideally, measured osmolarity should be determined on the same plasma sample that provides the [Na$^+$], [glucose], and [urea] values used to determine calculated osmolarity. Also, it's best to use the first venous blood sample drawn after the patient presents, since less time will have passed for methanol and ethylene glycol to be metabolized to organic acid anions, which do not show up in the osmolar gap. If you didn't think to request a measured osmolarity when first sending the blood sample to the lab (say, you didn't suspect a toxin until the lab reported a low Total CO$_2$), call the lab to see if they can add the test. Many labs refrigerate and retain blood samples for up to a week, allowing for add-on tests well after the initial assays are reported to you.

Check Eyes

Check the eyes carefully by both history and physical exam. Methanol is toxic to the optic nerve, so *blurred vision or blindness* in an inebriated patient suggests methanol intoxication. A fundoscopic exam may reveal abnormalities such as *retinal edema* or *hyperemia.*

Urinary Oxalate Crystals

Check a centrifuged urine sample for calcium oxalate crystals. These crystals strongly suggest ethylene glycol intoxication (p. 77) but a urine negative for these crystals does <u>not</u> rule out ethylene glycol. For images of these crystals, search on-line for "urine crystals ethylene glycol." Because calcium oxalate precipitates in many tissues, the total amount of calcium removed from body fluids can be large, sometimes causing hypocalcemia (low plasma $[Ca^{2+}]$) and resulting in seizures, arrhythmias, or coma.

Urinary Fluorescence

If you think that ingestion of radiator antifreeze solution (an important potential source of ethylene glycol ingestion) is a possibility, try to obtain an ultraviolet lamp (a.k.a. U.V., Wood's lamp, or black light). Many radiator solutions have a fluorescent dye (such as fluorescein) added to help auto mechanics detect radiator leaks. Pour some urine into an open container and see if it fluoresces under the lamp. The test works best within a few hours after ingestion. This test has limited sensitivity even during the first few hours, so a negative test does <u>not</u> rule out a radiator fluid ingestion. When using the U.V. light, don't leave the urine in a collection bag because the bag itself may fluoresce. Some paints and solvents also have fluorescent dyes in them, which can also cause urine to fluoresce following ingestion, so fluorescence does not automatically point to radiator fluid.

Treatment Concepts

In this and the following three chapters, I briefly introduce some key treatment concepts. Understanding these concepts will give you a foundation for working with therapeutic manuals and other detailed treatment resources and guidelines.

The first and most important step in treating metabolic acidosis is to identify and appropriately treat the *underlying condition*, that is, to remove the *cause* of the metabolic acidosis. Once this is done, you can consider the less important question of whether to directly raise the low plasma $[HCO_3^-]$ by giving the patient bicarbonate (or a "bicarbonate precursor" such as citrate, which is metabolized to bicarbonate by the liver). Treatment of the underlying conditions is beyond the scope of this book. The following paragraphs give you an introduction to bicarbonate therapy. As you'll see, the approach to bicarbonate is different in patients with organic vs. inorganic forms of metabolic acidosis.

When patients have *organic acidoses* (ketoacidosis, lactic acidosis), the decision of whether to give bicarbonate is complex and controversial. Bicarbonate is most likely to be considered in two circumstances: (1) if the acidemia is very severe and thought to be truly life threatening or (2) if the patient—especially a debilitated patient—is judged to be at high risk of developing ventilatory muscle fatigue from sustained, intense compensatory hyperventilation in response to the acidemia. The potential benefit in these situations is clear enough, but weighing against them are a number of factors, including: (1) Organic anions (lactate, acetoacetate, beta-hydroxybutyrate) in the body fluids can be metabolized to bicarbonate once the underlying condition is effectively treated, thus increasing plasma

$[HCO_3^-]$ without the use of supplemental bicarbonate. Giving extra bicarbonate can ultimately cause $[HCO_3^-]$ to rise too high, causing metabolic alkalosis (**"overshoot metabolic alkalosis"**); (2) Although giving bicarbonate makes sense physiologically, there is no clear evidence that doing so actually improves the outcome in patients with organic acidoses; (3) In patients with lactic acidosis, it is possible that giving bicarbonate stimulates additional lactic acid production and worsens the patient's condition. (4) In children with DKA, there is some evidence that giving bicarbonate may increase the risk of cerebral edema, which can be fatal. Other concerns, which we won't explore here, have also been raised.

So, to give or not give bicarbonate?—that is the question. Often, there is no simple answer. But as a practical matter, bicarbonate is sometimes given when a patient with ongoing *lactic acidosis*, such as from unresolved shock, has severe acidemia. In this situation, there is no consensus about how low pH should be allowed to fall before bicarbonate is considered, but most guidelines call for waiting until pH falls below 7.1 or even 7.0 (though picking a single pH is really quite arbitrary). In contrast, in *diabetic ketoacidosis*, bicarbonate is almost never given because treatment with i.v. insulin usually leads to a rapid improvement of the metabolic acidosis, since insulin effectively promotes the metabolism of the circulating ketoanions. In particular, in children with DKA, bicarbonate is not given because of concern about cerebral edema.

The situation is somewhat different in *inorganic* acidoses—those metabolic acidoses (e.g., diarrhea, renal failure, RTA) that are *not* normally associated with organic anion production. Here, bicarbonate is given more freely. In these patients, the risk of administering bicarbonate is usually low. In addition, the inorganic anions (e.g., Cl^-) cannot be metabolized to bicarbonate. Thus, there is no risk of overshoot metabolic alkalosis. If the clinician does not give bicarbonate to these patients, plasma $[HCO_3^-]$ will rise only very gradually, over a period of days, due to the slow process of renal bicarbonate regeneration. If bicarbonate losses are ongoing (e.g., during persistent diarrhea), bicarbonate may be needed to keep up with losses and stabilize plasma $[HCO_3^-]$. When metabolic acidosis is due to renal disease (renal failure, RTA), renal bicarbonate regeneration may be impaired, so $[HCO_3^-]$ may remain low indefinitely unless bicarbonate is given.*

Chronic metabolic acidosis (e.g., from chronic renal failure or RTA) has several specific adverse consequences. These include (1) buffering of carbonate and other bases in bones, which results in bone loss; (2) the breakdown of skeletal muscle, leading to muscle wasting and muscle weakness; and (3) impaired albumin syn-

---

*__Clinical note.__ One potential risk of giving bicarbonate in patients with inorganic acidosis pertains to potassium. If large amounts of bicarbonate are given, especially if infused rapidly, plasma $[HCO_3^-]$ can rise sharply, creating a steep downhill gradient for bicarbonate to move from the ECF into cells. As bicarbonate enters cells, extracellular K^+ is carried along to maintain electroneutrality, lowering plasma $[K^+]$. In patients who have a normal or, especially, a low plasma $[K^+]$ before treatment (recall that diarrhea and some types of RTA typically present with hypokalemia), this further reduction in $[K^+]$ can potentially result in severe hypokalemia, causing cardiac arrhythmias. Thus, in normokalemic (normal $[K^+]$) and, especially, hypokalemic patients, bicarbonate is usually given slowly and in conjunction with, or after, a period of potassium repletion.

thesis, resulting in low plasma [albumin]. Also (4), in patients with chronic kidney disease, the acidosis itself—that is, the low plasma [HCO_3^-]—leads to more rapid deterioration of renal function. All these adverse chronic effects are alleviated by giving either bicarbonate or "bicarbonate-precursors" such as citrate.

Summary

Metabolic acidosis is a disease process that decreases plasma [HCO_3^-], thereby causing acidemia. Any marked decline in plasma [HCO_3^-]—aside from that caused by compensation for respiratory alkalosis—is by definition metabolic acidosis. The four most common clinical causes of metabolic acidosis are: (1) diarrhea; (2) organic acidosis—lactic acidosis and ketoacidosis; (3) poisoning—especially with methanol, ethylene glycol, or salicylates (which also causes respiratory alkalosis); and (4) renal defects—renal failure or renal tubular acidosis (RTA). Specific lab tests include plasma lactate (lactic acidosis); creatinine and BUN (renal failure, RTA); ketones, glucose, and beta-hydroxybutyrate (ketoacidosis); and specific assays for methanol, ethylene glycol, and salicylate, as well as the osmolar gap. Treatment focuses on repairing the underlying disorder. The decision of whether to give bicarbonate is usually of secondary importance; it is also controversial for the organic acidoses.

Chapter 7

Metabolic Alkalosis

In this chapter, we'll study metabolic alkalosis in detail, focusing on its pathophysiology and on the clinical conditions that bring metabolic alkalosis about. Towards the end of the chapter, we'll also discuss some laboratory tests and treatment concepts relevant to metabolic alkalosis. As a reminder, metabolic alkalosis is defined as a disease process that increases plasma bicarbonate concentration, thereby producing alkalemia. Any marked increase in plasma $[HCO_3^-]$—aside from that arising as the compensation for a respiratory acidosis—is by definition metabolic alkalosis.*

Metabolic alkalosis is usually accompanied by hypokalemia. The low $[HCO_3^-]$, alone or in conjunction with low $[K^+]$, can produce three main types of adverse effects. First, especially when pH is above 7.6, treatment-refractory cardiac arrhythmias can occur. Second, the compensatory response for metabolic alkalosis is hypoventilation, which not only increases PCO_2 but also lowers arterial PO_2. As a result, especially in patients with pre-existing impairments of gas exchange due to lung disease, tissue oxygen delivery may be reduced. Contributing to this effect, alkalemia reduces hemoglobin's ability to unload oxygen at the tissues. Third, metabolic alkalosis sometimes causes neurological and neuromuscular impairments, including malaise, lethargy, and weakness. Less commonly, the following can also occur: agitation, confusion, stupor, muscle twitching, tetany, seizures, and coma.

To understand how metabolic alkalosis occurs clinically, it's useful to begin with some key concepts.

Key Concepts:
Threshold, Generation, and Maintenance

If excess bicarbonate enters the ECF, the kidney—as part of its normal, regulatory function—excretes the excess in the urine, thus holding plasma $[HCO_3^-]$ relatively constant. To understand how this happens, it's useful to think of the kidney as having a **threshold level** for bicarbonate. I'll explain this concept with reference to situations you are already familiar with and then show how it applies to the kidney. Scan the two following figures, then keep reading:

---

*Terminology.** The term metabolic alkalosis is introduced and fully explained in Chapter 2. For a quick refresher of the main point, see the illustration on page 28. The concept of compensation is explained in Chapter 5.

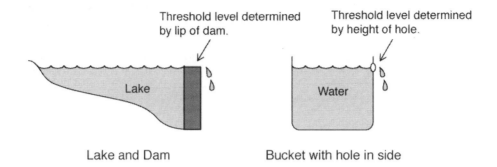

Lake and Dam Bucket with hole in side

In these figures, notice that some specific characteristic of each structure—the lip of the dam and the hole in the bucket—sets a maximum above which the water level cannot rise. Once water starts to exceed that level, it starts to spill, so the water level cannot rise further. The maximum water level permitted by the structure is the threshold level. Of course, if for some reason, the lip or hole rises, the water level can rise, too. By analogy to these physical structures, the kidney is sometimes said to have thresholds for particular substances in the plasma. If the plasma concentration of one of these substances starts to rise above its renal threshold level, the substance starts to spill into the urine, thus curtailing the increase in its plasma level. In effect, the existence of a renal threshold places a cap, or ceiling, on the plasma concentration—skimming off and excreting whatever exceeds the threshold. For bicarbonate, the threshold is usually around 25 mmol/liter, with a fair amount of variation among individuals. Plasma levels much above this threshold result in the urinary spillage of large amounts of bicarbonate. The existence of this threshold helps explain why plasma $[HCO_3^-]$ is normally close to 25 mmol/l.

The spillage of excess bicarbonate occurs by two mechanisms. First, as plasma $[HCO_3^-]$ rises, the amount of bicarbonate filtered at the glomerulus increases (since Amount of Bicarbonate Filtered = Volume of Fluid Filtered x Concentration of Bicarbonate in Fluid). The renal tubule is limited in how much bicarbonate it can reabsorb, so excess filtered bicarbonate is not efficiently returned to the blood. Thus, some filtered bicarbonate remains in the tubular fluid and is excreted in the urine. Second, special cells in the collecting duct called **beta-intercalated cells** (a.k.a. B-type intercalated cells) have the ability to *secrete* excess bicarbonate into the tubular fluid; this secreted bicarbonate is excreted in the urine.* Though these two mechanisms are quite different at the cellular level, the end result is the same: excess bicarbonate is excreted in the urine and plasma $[HCO_3^-]$ is prevented from rising. Of the two mechanisms, the limitation on reabsorption was discovered first. For this reason, the renal threshold was originally known as a "reabsorptive threshold," and this term is often still used.

All this leads to a question: If the kidney normally spills excess plasma bicarbonate into the urine, how is it even possible for metabolic alkalosis (a rise in

---

*__Reminder.__ *Secretion* refers to the entry of substances *into* the nephron lumen, whereas *reabsorption* refers to the movement of substances *out of* the nephron lumen. For a review of basic renal physiology and terminology, see the start of Chapter 4.

[HCO$_3^-$]) to occur? The answer is that many of the clinical conditions that add bicarbonate to the body fluids have the *additional* effect of producing various electrolyte and other abnormalities, and some of these additional abnormalities *act on the kidney to raise its bicarbonate threshold level.* With the threshold level raised, more bicarbonate can accumulate in plasma, making it possible for metabolic alkalosis to occur. The most important of these threshold-raising abnormalities are: **volume depletion, chloride depletion, hypokalemia,** and **aldosterone excess.** I'll say more about these four abnormalities in a moment, but for now it's enough to know that if one or more of them is present, the bicarbonate threshold increases.

It follows from these points that, when you consider a patient with metabolic alkalosis, you have to think about *both* (1) processes that add bicarbonate to the body fluids and (2) processes that raise the kidney's bicarbonate threshold. These two sets of processes are described with a particular terminology. Processes that add bicarbonate to the plasma are said to **generate** the metabolic alkalosis. Processes or factors that raise the threshold, and thus cause the body to retain (i.e., not excrete) the newly generated bicarbonate, are said to **maintain** the metabolic alkalosis. When both generation and maintenance are present, metabolic alkalosis develops:

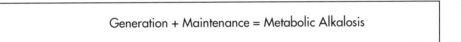

Generation + Maintenance = Metabolic Alkalosis

To better understand these concepts, study this figure, then refer back to it as you continue to read:

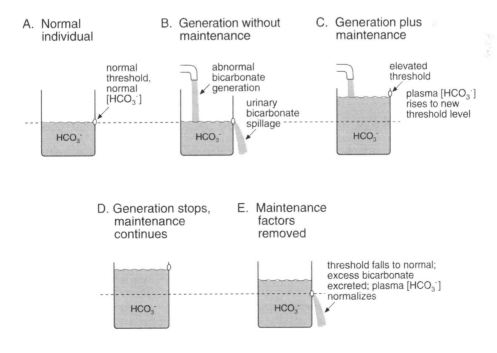

89

Bucket A represents a normal individual. There is no abnormal bicarbonate generation and the renal threshold is normal. Bucket B represents generation without maintenance. Excess bicarbonate is produced and enters the ECF, but the threshold is normal, so the bicarbonate spills into the urine without a marked increase in plasma [HCO_3^-] occurring. Bucket C represents generation plus maintenance. Excess bicarbonate is produced and retained, thus increasing plasma [HCO_3^-]. No bicarbonate spills unless [HCO_3^-] reaches the new threshold level. This patient has metabolic alkalosis. Note that if [HCO_3^-] does reach the new threshold level, bicarbonate starts to spill and [HCO_3^-] is maintained at the new (higher) level. Bucket D shows what happens to Bucket C if generation stops but the factors maintaining the abnormal threshold remain. Plasma [HCO_3^-] stays high. That is, metabolic alkalosis persists. Only after the factors that maintain the alkalosis are removed does the threshold fall. At that point, the kidney can excrete excess bicarbonate, correcting the metabolic alkalosis, as shown in Bucket E.

Raising the Bicarbonate Threshold: Four Maintenance Factors

As mentioned, four abnormalities—which I'll call "maintenance factors"—can raise the renal threshold for bicarbonate, thereby impairing the urinary spillage of excess bicarbonate, letting plasma [HCO_3^-] rise, and helping maintain metabolic alkalosis. The four factors are:

1. Volume Depletion
2. Chloride Depletion
3. Hypokalemia
4. Aldosterone Excess*

Let's see how these four factors raise the threshold. We'll approach this topic in two ways: general and specific.

General Explanation. We've already seen that the kidney's normal bicarbonate threshold (roughly 25 mmol/l) exists for two reasons: a limit to the tubule's bicarbonate-reabsorbing capacity, and the existence of a mechanism that secretes excess bicarbonate. It follows that the four maintenance factors must operate by either increasing the rate of bicarbonate reabsorption or decreasing the rate of bicarbonate secretion—and, in fact, all the maintenance factors operate through one or both of these routes. This is the general explanation, and for most clinical purposes it's all you need to know. (If you don't want more details right now, feel free to skip directly to the heading on page 93, "Two Maintenance Factors Also Help Generate Alkalosis.")

*****Mnemonic.** HAVoC—Hypokalemia, Aldosterone, Volume, Chloride. This mnemonic makes physiologic sense since these factors actually do cause some havoc by maintaining metabolic alkalosis. In the text, I list volume and chloride depletion first because they are usually the most important.

Specific Explanation. At the cellular level, each of the four maintenance factors works through several different mechanisms. These mechanisms tend to be complex and not fully understood, so it's not worth studying all of them. But we will look at a few important ones, to give you a sense of the processes involved. Before starting, take a moment to review the figure on page 49 to remind yourself how and where protons are secreted, and how proton secretion and bicarbonate reabsorption both arise from the $CO_2 + H_2O \rightarrow HCO_3^- + H^+$ reaction inside renal tubular cells.[*]

1. Volume Depletion

Recall that total body stores of Na^+ is a crucial determinant of ECF volume. During volume depletion, to help prevent ECF volume from falling even further, the kidneys work to minimize the urinary spillage of Na^+. The kidneys do this by increasing the reabsorption of filtered Na^+ in both the proximal and distal nephron. In the proximal tubule, much of the Na^+ reabsorption occurs via an $Na^+- H^+$ exchanger—so, as Na^+ reabsorption increases, H^+ secretion increases too. Since H^+ secretion and HCO_3^- reabsorption make use of the same intracellular reaction $(CO_2 + H_2O \rightarrow HCO_3^- + H^+)$, bicarbonate reabsorption increases as well, thus raising the plasma bicarbonate threshold. In the distal nephron, specifically in the collecting duct, Na^+ reabsorption leads to increased proton secretion by an indirect route. To understand this route, study this figure, then keep reading:

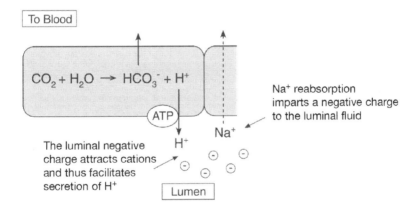

In the collecting duct, plasma aldosterone, which is elevated due to volume depletion, stimulates renal tubular cells to reabsorb Na^+ from the luminal fluid.[**] Because Na^+ is positively charged, its reabsorption imparts a slight negative charge to luminal fluid in the collecting duct. This negative charge electrically attracts H^+ and thus facilitates proton secretion, which is carried out by the H^+–ATPase.

---

[*]**Hint.** To understand the specific mechanisms discussed here, you need a good grasp of how bicarbonate reabsorption works. If you don't already have one, review Chapter 4, paying special attention to the explanations of bicarbonate reabsorption (pp. 42–43) and proton secretion (p. 48–50).

[**]**Reminder.** The kidneys sense and respond to volume depletion by releasing renin into the plasma. This renin release is the first step in the renin-angiotensin-aldosterone cascade, the final step of which is the release of aldosterone by the adrenal cortex.

Because this mechanism operates through the creation of an electrical charge, which attracts protons to the lumen, it is sometimes described as the "voltage-dependent facilitation of proton secretion." In addition, by another mechanism, the elevated plasma aldosterone directly stimulates the H^+–ATPase. As in the proximal tubule, increased H^+ secretion translates into increased HCO_3^- reabsorption and, therefore, an elevated HCO_3^- threshold.

2. Chloride Depletion

Many of the same clinical problems (e.g., vomiting, discussed later in the chapter) that cause volume depletion also cause chloride to be lost from the body. Chloride depletion and volume depletion act together as follows. When Cl^- is lost, plasma $[Cl^-]$ falls. Since luminal fluid derives from the filtration of plasma, luminal $[Cl^-]$ in the proximal tubule falls as well. Some of the Na^+ that is reabsorbed from the proximal tubule, in response to volume depletion, is reabsorbed along with Cl^- to balance the positive charge on the Na^+; this reabsorption of Cl^- lowers luminal $[Cl^-]$ even further. Thus, by the time luminal fluid reaches the collecting duct, its $[Cl^-]$ is *very* low. To see what happens next, scan this figure, then keep reading:

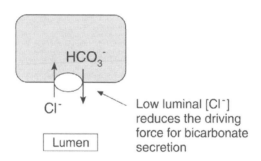

As mentioned earlier in the chapter, a special group of cells in the collecting duct (beta-intercalated cells) help keep plasma $[HCO_3^-]$ in the normal range by secreting excess bicarbonate. This secretion is carried out by Cl^-–HCO_3^- exchangers located in the cell's luminal membrane; these exchangers reabsorb Cl^- while secreting HCO_3^-. Normally, the influx of Cl^- from the lumen into the cell is steeply "downhill" (i.e., $[Cl^-]$ is much higher in the lumen than in the cell) and thus provides a driving force for Cl^-–HCO_3^- exchange. However, when luminal $[Cl^-]$ is very low, as it is during chloride depletion, the driving force is reduced and bicarbonate secretion slows. Thus, some of the excess plasma bicarbonate that would otherwise be eliminated by the kidney is retained in the body.

3. Hypokalemia

In the collecting duct, an ATP-powered H^+–K^+ exchanger can secrete protons while reabsorbing K^+ from the luminal fluid, as shown here:

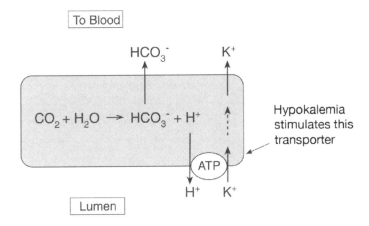

Hypokalemia stimulates this exchanger; this makes physiological sense since the reabsorption of K^+ keeps plasma $[K^+]$ from falling further. But in the process of reabsorbing K^+, this transporter secretes H^+ and, as a result, HCO_3^- reabsorption increases—again raising the plasma threshold for bicarbonate.

4. Aldosterone excess

Plasma aldosterone levels can rise in two ways. Most commonly, plasma [aldosterone] increases because of volume depletion (see footnote p. 91). Less commonly, a defect in the adrenal cortex itself (e.g., an adrenal adenoma) causes autonomous aldosterone secretion. In either case, the high plasma [aldosterone] stimulates bicarbonate reabsorption in the collecting duct by the same mechanisms discussed above for volume depletion. The result, once again, is an elevated bicarbonate threshold.

Two Maintenance Factors Also Help Generate Alkalosis

As we've seen, four factors (volume depletion, chloride depletion, hypokalemia, and aldosterone excess) impair the urinary spillage of excess bicarbonate and thus can maintain metabolic alkalosis—hence the term "maintenance factors." However, two of the four maintenance factors, aldosterone excess and hypokalemia, have an additional effect: they stimulate the kidney to *regenerate* bicarbonate. That is, they stimulate the kidney to produce *new* bicarbonate, which is added to the ECF. As a reminder, recall that whereas bicarbonate *reabsorption* merely returns filtered bicarbonate to the blood, and thus cannot raise plasma $[HCO_3^-]$ above its current level, bicarbonate *regeneration* can actually increase plasma $[HCO_3^-]$. By stimulating bicarbonate regeneration, aldosterone excess and hypokalemia can thus contribute to the *generation* of metabolic alkalosis, as well as to its maintenance.

How do hypokalemia and aldosterone excess stimulate bicarbonate regeneration? During hypokalemia, the low $[K^+]$ of the ECF creates a downhill gradient for intracellular K^+ to move out of cells—a so-called "cellular shift" of K^+ from ICF to ECF. To balance the positive charge on this shifted K^+, some HCO_3^- also moves from ICF to ECF. This bicarbonate shift lowers intracellular $[HCO_3^-]$ and, as a result, intracellular pH decreases. The low intracellular pH stimulates ammonium excretion, which is the main route for regenerating bicarbonate. In essence, the cell "thinks" the low intracellular pH is caused by metabolic acidosis, so it responds "appropriately" by regenerating new bicarbonate to raise plasma $[HCO_3^-]$. Because elevated plasma [aldosterone] promotes urinary K^+ excretion, it can lead to hypokalemia and thus stimulate ammonium excretion by the same mechanism just described.

In the next section, we'll see how the four maintenance factors come into play during the clinical conditions that cause metabolic alkalosis.*

Diseases that Cause Metabolic Alkalosis

Metabolic alkalosis develops in four main clinical settings:

1. Loss of gastric fluid—vomiting or nasogastric drainage
2. Diuretic therapy—especially when used to treat edema
3. Mechanical ventilation of patients with chronic respiratory acidosis
4. "Volume-resistant" causes of metabolic alkalosis

Let's consider these four clinical settings individually.

Loss of Gastric Fluid

The following figure may look familiar, since it is the same one presented in Chapter 6. It applies here as well. Study the figure again, then refer to it as you continue to read:

---

*__Clinical note.__ Perhaps surprisingly, patients with renal failure, which normally causes metabolic *acidosis* (p. 77), are especially prone to developing metabolic *alkalosis* if a separate clinical problem (e.g., vomiting, discussed shortly in the text) rapidly generates excess bicarbonate. Here's why. During renal failure, metabolic acidosis arises because the damaged kidney cannot regenerate all bicarbonate that is lost while buffering the normal daily load of endogenously produced acids (p. 47, 78). Because endogenous acid production is typically only about 70 mmols H^+ per day, the onset of acidosis is gradual. This gradual acidotic process can easily get obscured if abnormal quantities of bicarbonate are rapidly added to the body fluids. At the same time, low GFR from the renal failure helps maintain the alkalosis, as follows. Low GFR means little bicarbonate is filtered, and the small filtered load makes it easier for the renal tubules to reabsorb all the bicarbonate—so there is a tendency for bicarbonate reabsorption to be complete (i.e., no urinary spillage) even when plasma $[HCO_3^-]$ is elevated. If you want, you can think of low GFR as a fifth maintenance factor. This GFR mechanism can also come into play during volume depletion, which, when severe, reduces GFR.

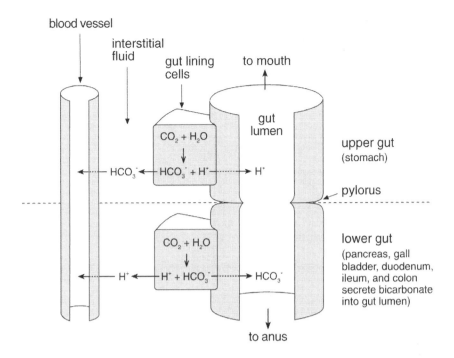

Under normal conditions—especially following a meal (postprandial)—protons are secreted into the stomach lumen. Proton secretion may be so rapid postprandially that the pH of stomach contents falls to 1.0 (an [H^+] of 100 mmol/l). Notice in the figure that these protons are produced in cells lining the stomach by the reaction $CO_2 + H_2O \rightarrow HCO_3^- + H^+$. This means that protons and bicarbonate are produced in equal quantities. The bicarbonate enters the blood. The result is that when stomach contents are acidified, plasma [HCO_3^-] rises very slightly.

Normally, even this minimal rise in plasma [HCO_3^-] is temporary. The reason is that the passage of stomach contents into the duodenum stimulates the pancreas to secrete bicarbonate-rich fluids into the gut lumen. As shown in the figure, the production of this pancreatic bicarbonate adds protons to the blood. These protons consume plasma bicarbonate ($H^+ + HCO_3^- \rightarrow CO_2 + H_2O$). Thus, under normal conditions, bicarbonate added to blood by the stomach is eliminated due to the subsequent actions of the pancreas. The end result is that plasma [HCO_3^-] and pH are unchanged.

However, when vomiting or nasogastric drainage are present, stomach contents, which exit the body via the mouth or nasogastric tube, do not enter the duodenum and thus do not stimulate the pancreas to secrete its bicarbonate-rich fluids into the gut lumen. Thus, bicarbonate added to blood by the stomach is not matched by protons added to the blood from the pancreas. As a result, there is a net addition of bicarbonate to the blood. Plasma [HCO_3^-] starts to rise, and it continues to rise if vomiting or nasogastric drainage persists. That sequence of events represents the *generation* of the metabolic alkalosis—the addition of net bicarbonate to the ECF. *Maintenance*—the raising of the renal threshold for bicarbonate—occurs in three steps:

<u>First</u>, gastric fluid contains (in addition to protons) water, sodium, chloride, and a small amount of potassium. As a result, when gastric fluid is lost through vomiting or nasogastric drainage, some depletion of volume, chloride, and potassium occurs. These depletions all act as maintenance factors, as described earlier in the chapter.

<u>Second</u>, these depletions (maintenance factors) are initially mild, so they do not completely prevent excess plasma bicarbonate from spilling in the urine. The bicarbonate (an anion) that does spill attracts and carries along Na^+ and K^+ (cations) in the urine, maintaining electroneutrality of the urine. These ions also act osmotically to carry additional water into the urine. The additional urinary losses of Na^+, K^+, and water exacerbate both the volume depletion and hypokalemia. The maintenance factors are now becoming more significant.

<u>Third</u>, the worsening volume depletion is detected by the kidney, resulting in the activation of the renin-angiotensin-aldosterone system, which raises plasma [aldosterone]. Aldosterone itself is a maintenance factor. In addition, aldosterone stimulates the kidney to secrete K^+, leading to further potassium losses. At this point, significant volume and chloride depletion, as well as hypokalemia and aldosterone excess, are present. These factors maintain the metabolic alkalosis even if the vomiting or gastric drainage stops. Only when the maintenance factors are corrected can the excess bicarbonate be excreted.

Diuretic Therapy

The treatment of edema with thiazide or loop diuretics is a common cause of metabolic alkalosis.* Both the generation and maintenance of this alkalosis can be understood by considering three topics:

1. Contraction alkalosis. In patients with edema, diuretics can reduce ECF volume by five or more liters. Thiazide and loop diuretics promote the excretion of Na^+, Cl^-, and water, but not bicarbonate. Therefore, almost all the bicarbonate originally present in the excreted edema fluid is retained in the body. Because fluid is lost, the bicarbonate is distributed in a smaller ECF volume, so plasma $[HCO_3^-]$ rises. This process is called contraction alkalosis because the ECF seems to "contract" around a fixed amount of bicarbonate. The following figure illustrates this process with sample numbers:

***Clinical note.** Heart failure, nephrotic syndrome, and liver cirrhosis with ascites are the three most common conditions that result in edema and are treated with diuretics.

Before diuretic therapy
ECF expanded, edematous

After diuretic therapy
ECF 'contracted' by loss of saline

ECF Volume = 19 liters

Total ECF bicarbonate = 456 mmol

$[HCO_3^-] = 456/19 = 24$ mmol/l

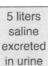

ECF Volume = 14 liters

Total ECF bicarbonate = 456 mmol

$[HCO_3^-] = 456/14 = 32.6$ mmol/l

5 liters
saline
excreted
in urine

2. Volume and chloride depletion. In patients with edema, a substantial fraction of extracellular fluid is "third spaced," meaning that it is localized to the sub-cutaneous tissues, peritoneal cavity, or other potential spaces (e.g., the pleural or pericardial cavities). This third-spaced ECF fluid forms a partially isolated fluid compartment that has limited effect on fluid dynamics in the body. Thus, even though *total* ECF volume (the sum of normal ECF + third-spaced fluid) may be expanded in patients with edema, the portion of ECF volume that is not third-spaced, including plasma volume, is often depleted. These patients are said to have *effective volume depletion*, since the physiological consequences (including increased bicarbonate reabsorption by the kidney) are the same as in ordinary volume depletion.* This effective volume depletion is exacerbated by diuretic therapy, which removes both third-spaced and non-third spaced volume. At the same time, the loss of chloride in the urine depletes body stores of chloride. Effective volume depletion and chloride depletion both help maintain the alkalosis.

3. Aldosterone excess and hypokalemia. Volume depletion caused by diuretics stimulates the renin-angiotensin-aldosterone system, raising plasma [aldosterone]. Since aldosterone promotes K^+ secretion by the kidney, the elevated [aldosterone] can cause hypokalemia. The combination of aldosterone excess and hypokalemia helps maintain the metabolic alkalosis.

Mechanical Ventilation of Patients with Chronic Respiratory Acidosis

The patient with chronic respiratory acidosis has high plasma $[HCO_3^-]$ due to renal compensation. If this patient deteriorates and must be placed on a mechanical ventilator, and this mechanical ventilation rapidly reduces PCO_2 to normal or near normal levels, $[HCO_3^-]$ will remain elevated. The patient now has high $[HCO_3^-]$ and normal PCO_2—by definition, an uncompensated metabolic alkalosis. This

---

* **Terminology.** Sometimes the term "effective *circulating* volume depletion" is used to emphasize the fact that third-spaced ECF volume cannot freely enter the vasculature and thus does not readily circulate.

condition is often called **post-hypercapnic metabolic alkalosis.** This situation arises most often in patients with hypercapnia* from COPD who experience an acute worsening of their condition (say, due to an acute lung infection) and require mechanical ventilation. The sequence looks like this:

Step 1:	Step 2:	Step 3:	Step 4:	
Respiratory acidosis	→ Compensatory rise in plasma $[HCO_3^-]$	→ Mechanical ventilation lowers PCO_2	→ $[HCO_3^-]$ remains elevated	= Metabolic Alkalosis

This sequence generates the alkalosis. Two factors maintain it:

> First, in chronic respiratory acidosis, the high PCO_2 stimulates renal tubular cells to increase bicarbonate reabsorption, raising the bicarbonate threshold and thus maintaining the elevated $[HCO_3^-]$. Although the decrease in PCO_2 that results from mechanical ventilation removes the stimulus, there appears to be a "memory" effect whereby reabsorption remains high for another 24 hours or so. During this period, the metabolic alkalosis is maintained.

> Second, patients with chronic lung disease like COPD often have other problems (e.g., hypertension, cor pulmonale) that are treated with low-salt diets and diuretics. These treatments deplete volume, chloride, and sometimes potassium. In such patients, metabolic alkalosis can be maintained indefinitely unless the electrolyte deficits are replaced.

Volume-Resistant Causes of Metabolic Alkalosis

Taken together, the conditions that have just been discussed (gastric fluid loss, diuretics, post-hypercapnia) account for roughly 95 percent of cases of metabolic alkalosis. In all these situations, the alkalosis is maintained largely by deficits of volume and chloride. (Hypokalemia and aldosterone excess usually play a less important role.) These deficits can be corrected by giving the patient volume-expanding (NaCl-containing) fluids. Once these deficits are corrected, the kidney can excrete the excess bicarbonate, which resolves the metabolic alkalosis. Therefore, the causes of metabolic alkalosis we've considered so far are sometimes referred to, as a group, using the umbrella term **volume-responsive metabolic alkalosis**—that is, the alkalosis "responds" to treatment with volume-expanding fluids.

In contrast, there exists a group of uncommon causes of metabolic alkalosis, together comprising about 5 percent of cases, which arise through different mechanisms that cannot be reversed by giving the patient volume-expanding fluids. These are referred to with the umbrella term **volume-resistant metabolic**

---

*__Terminology.__ The word root *cap* refers to carbon dioxide. Hypercapnia refers to a PCO_2 above the normal range. Hypocapnia refers to a sub-normal PCO_2. Normocapnia refers to a PCO_2 in the normal range. The term post-hypercapnic indicates "after hypercapnia."

alkalosis—because the alkalosis "resists" (does not respond to) treatment with volume-expanding fluids. We'll consider these volume-resistant causes now.[*]

The most common example of volume-resistant metabolic alkalosis is **primary hyperaldosteronism**. In this condition, an intrinsic adrenal problem, usually an **adrenal adenoma** or **adrenal hyperplasia**, causes the adrenal gland to oversecrete aldosterone. The elevated plasma [aldosterone] acts on the kidney to promote urinary K^+ excretion, causing hypokalemia. The combination of aldosterone excess and hypokalemia is responsible for both generating and maintaining the alkalosis. The elevated [aldosterone] also promotes Na^+ reabsorption by the kidney. Thus, Na^+ reabsorption increases *even though volume depletion is not present*. This high Na^+ reabsorption, when occurring along with ongoing dietary intake of sodium and water, expands ECF volume, and with it plasma volume. As a result, blood pressure tends to increase. Therefore, patients with primary hyperaldosteronism generally present with **hypertension**. This situation contrasts with the volume-responsive causes of metabolic alkalosis, which are associated with volume depletion and usually present with either **normal blood pressure or orthostatic hypotension**.

Thinking about primary hyperaldosteronism helps you understand a number of other causes of volume-resistant metabolic alkalosis. For example, **ACTH-secreting tumors** of the pituitary gland cause abnormally high levels of ACTH, which stimulates the adrenals to secrete aldosterone, again raising plasma [aldosterone] levels.[**] In **Cushing's syndrome**, which is characterized by high cortisol levels, the cortisol has some mineralocorticoid (aldosterone-like) effects on the kidney—so the body acts as though there is a primary elevation in aldosterone. Likewise, **licorice** (real licorice, not artificially flavored) has mineralocorticoid effects; it can cause mild metabolic alkalosis if consumed in sufficient quantities. In these last two conditions (Cushings, licorice overconsumption) the body acts as if aldosterone is elevated, but unlike in primary hyperaldosteronism and ACTH-secreting tumors, actual plasma aldosterone levels are usually low or low-normal (because there is "feedback inhibition" of aldosterone production due to the presence of an aldosterone agonist). In **renal artery stenosis**, the arterial stenosis (narrowing) impairs renal blood flow, and the kidney responds just as it would if blood flow were reduced due to volume depletion—that is, the renin-angiotensin-aldosterone system is activated and plasma [aldosterone] rises; in essence, the kidney "thinks" volume is depleted. As with primary hyperaldosteronism, all these conditions expand ECF volume and thus usually present with hypertension.

Two interesting but rare genetic causes of volume-resistant metabolic alkalosis are **Bartter syndrome** (pronounced "barter") and **Gitelman syndrome**. In these conditions, genetic defects in the renal tubule's ion transporters lead to high urinary spillage of Na^+, Cl^-, and K^+. The effect is much the same as would occur

---

[*] **Terminology**. Instead of "volume responsive" and "volume resistant," some texts and clinicians use "saline responsive" and "saline resistant," or "chloride responsive" and "chloride resistant." These pairs of terms have essentially the same meaning and can be used interchangeably.

[**] **Reminder.** As its name suggests, adrenocorticotropic hormone (ACTH), which is produced by the anterior pituitary gland, stimulates the adrenal cortex, which produces both corticosteroids and aldosterone.

if a diuretic were continually active. The resulting depletions of volume, chloride, and potassium, and the rise in plasma aldosterone that occurs in response to volume depletion (due to activation of the renin-angiotensin-aldosterone system), generate and maintain the metabolic alkalosis. However, simply replacing electrolytes (say, by giving the patient NaCl or KCl) doesn't correct the alkalosis because the urinary loss of these ions is ongoing. In contrast to most other causes of volume-resistant metabolic alkalosis, Bartter and Gitelman syndromes are associated with volume depletion and thus do not present with hypertension; like the volume-responsive causes of metabolic alkalosis, they tend to present with either normal blood pressure or orthostatic hypotension.*

Potassium status in metabolic alkalosis. Metabolic alkalosis, both volume-responsive and volume-resistant, typically presents with hypokalemia. The reason is that [aldosterone] is elevated, either secondary to volume depletion (e.g., in vomiting) or as a primary defect (e.g., in primary hyperaldosteronism). In both cases, the elevated [aldosterone] promotes urinary K^+ excretion, leading to hypokalemia.

Specific Diagnostic Tests

As we have seen, the most common causes of metabolic alkalosis—vomiting, nasogastric drainage, diuretics, post-hypercapnic mechanical ventilation—are all associated with volume depletion. These causes of metabolic alkalosis are usually obvious from the clinical setting, occasionally aided by a urinary diuretic screen if you are concerned that diuretics are being used surreptitiously for weight loss. As a result, it is usually fairly easy to differentiate between the **volume-responsive** and **volume-resistant** causes: suspicion of a volume-resistant cause arises when a volume-responsive cause (vomiting, nasogastric drainage, diuretics, mechanical ventilation) is not obvious from the history and physical exam.

If a volume-resistant cause is suspected, it is useful to seek confirmation by measuring the *urine chloride concentration* or, if that is not available, the *urine sodium concentration*. (The urine [Cl^-] is a better test for this purpose, but not all hospitals offer it.) Here's the rationale. During volume depletion, filtered Na^+ and Cl^- both are strongly reabsorbed by the renal tubule as part of the kidney's attempt to maintain plasma volume. This reabsorption tends to lower urine [Na^+] and [Cl^-]. Thus, a low urine value (<15 mmol/l) for Na^+ or Cl^- implies the presence of volume depletion and points to a volume-responsive cause for the metabolic alkalosis. In contrast, a higher urine value (> 20–30 mmol/l) for Na^+ or Cl^- points to a normal or expanded ECF volume and thus suggests a volume-resistant cause for the metabolic alkalosis. The following box discusses the limitations of these urine tests and explains why the [Cl^-] test is better. If you're a first-time student of acid-base, you might want to skip this box for now to avoid getting bogged down in details.

---

*Going further.** Bartter and Gitelman syndromes affect ion transporters in characteristic locations in the nephron. Bartter syndrome affects the ascending limb of Henle's loop. It mimics the action of loop diuretics such as furosemide, which act on Henle's loop. In contrast, Gitelman syndrome affects the distal convoluted tubule (DCT). It mimics the action of thiazide diuretics, which act on the DCT. An additional, very rare genetic cause of volume-resistant metabolic alkalosis, which I won't discuss further, is Liddle syndrome.

Measuring Urine [Cl⁻] or [Na⁺] in Metabolic Alkalosis: Limitations to the Tests

Measuring urine $[Cl^-]$ or $[Na^+]$ can help you confirm whether a volume-resistant cause is responsible for metabolic alkalosis. However, these urine tests have limitations, which are especially pronounced for the Na^+ test. Knowing these limitations will help you interpret the test results more accurately.

First, current or recent diuretic use causes Na^+ and Cl^- to be excreted even when volume is depleted. Therefore, urine $[Na^+]$ and $[Cl^-]$ may not be low even during volume depletion. However, if you are concerned that the patient is not giving an accurate history about diuretic use, you can rule out diuretics with a urinary diuretic screen.

Second, the urine Na^+ test is not sensitive for volume depletion when bicarbonate is spilling into the urine. The problem is that bicarbonate (an anion) attracts and carries sodium (a cation) with it into the urine, raising urine $[Na^+]$ even during volume depletion. Typically, bicarbonate is spilled during metabolic alkalosis in three situations: (1) Early in the course of metabolic alkalosis. During this early phase, generation is in place but maintenance may not yet be fully active—so some of the newly produced bicarbonate gets excreted. (2) When additional vomiting or nasogastric drainage occurs after the metabolic alkalosis is already established. In this circumstance, the production of additional bicarbonate causes plasma $[HCO_3^-]$ to rise above the current threshold level, leading to urinary spillage. (3) When a patient with metabolic alkalosis receives sodium or chloride either intravenously (say, via an NaCl infusion, as might be used in the treatment of volume-responsive metabolic alkalosis—see "Treatment Concepts" later in the chapter) or orally by ingesting foods or beverages rich in sodium or chloride. Once maintenance factors start to be reversed by the sodium or chloride, the renal bicarbonate threshold starts to fall and previously retained bicarbonate begins to spill into the urine.

However, even when bicarbonate is spilling in the urine, urine $[Cl^-]$ remains low during volume depletion. For this reason urine $[Cl^-]$ is the preferred test. If your lab offers only the $[Na^+]$ test, keeping the above limitations in mind can help you identify those circumstances in which an elevated urine $[Na^+]$ is not suggestive of volume-resistant metabolic alkalosis.

Finally, if your lab offers only the urine $[Na^+]$ test, you can partly compensate for the above limitations by also measuring urine pH, ideally on the same urine sample. Here's the approach. Because bicarbonate (a base) in the urine raises pH, a urine pH above 7.0 suggests that bicarbonate spillage has occurred. In contrast, a urine pH below 6.5 suggests a relatively low urine $[HCO_3^-]$ and no marked bicarbonate spillage. Thus, if urinary $[Na^+]$ is not low, and urine pH is below 6.5, and you are confident that diuretics have not been used, a volume-resistant cause is likely.

The following table summarizes information useful for differentiating volume-responsive and volume-resistant causes of metabolic alkalosis. To reinforce some of the main points covered above, take a moment to review this table before continuing.

Diagnostic Summary: Volume-Responsive vs. Volume-Resistant Metabolic Alkalosis		
	Volume-Responsive	**Volume-Resistant**
Extracellular Volume	Low	High
Blood Pressure	Usually normal or orthostatic hypotension	Usually Hypertension
Urine [Cl⁻] and [Na⁺]	Low (< 15)	Not low (>20–30). Box in text gives fine points
Plasma [K⁺]	Low	Low
Most Common Causes	Vomiting, nasogastric drainage, diuretics, post-hypercapnic mechanical ventilation. These volume-responsive causes account for ~95% of cases of metabolic alkalosis. Specific cause usually obvious from clinical setting with exception of surreptitious diuretic use.	Primary hyperaldosteronism from adrenal adenoma or adrenal hyperplasia. Volume-resistant causes usually start to be considered when a volume-responsive cause is not obvious from the clinical setting.
Less Common and Rare Causes (partial list, not all discussed in text)	In adults: villous adenoma of the large bowel. In infants: congenital chloride diarrhea.	Cushing's syndrome, heavy consumption of real licorice, renal artery stenosis, ACTH-secreting tumors, renin-secreting tumors, adrenal carcinoma, and rare genetic conditions including Gitelman, Bartter, and Liddle syndromes.

Treatment Concepts

The **volume-responsive causes** of metabolic alkalosis are treated by repairing the underlying condition, when possible, and reversing the maintenance factors, as follows:

- *Volume depletion* is treated with volume-expanding fluids, typically normal saline (a.k.a. isotonic saline or 0.9 percent NaCl).
- *Hypokalemia* is treated by giving KCl as either oral supplements or, if necessary, through the cautious use of i.v. supplementation.

- *Chloride depletion* gets repaired when you treat volume depletion and hypokalemia, because the Na^+ and K^+ are given as NaCl and KCl.
- *Aldosterone excess* corrects itself once the volume depletion is repaired, since aldosterone is elevated secondary to volume depletion.

When **diuretics** cause the alkalosis, you cannot simply give volume-expanding fluids because doing so undercuts the therapeutically desirable volume depletion produced by the diuretics. Sometimes giving KCl and/or acetazolamide (Diamox) is effective. Acetazolamide is a mild diuretic that is a carbonic anhydrase (c.a.) inhibitor. Since c.a. plays a key role in bicarbonate reabsorption, inhibiting c.a. causes bicarbonate to spill into the urine, thus reducing plasma $[HCO_3^-]$. However, acetazolamide also causes rapid urinary spillage of potassium, so acetazolamide therapy must be accompanied by aggressive potassium supplementation. Other treatment options for patients with diuretic-induced metabolic alkalosis also exist. Treatment of **volume-resistant** causes involves repairing the underlying condition when possible, though various other measures (which are beyond the scope of this book) are also sometimes helpful.

In general, correcting metabolic alkalosis is especially urgent in two circumstances. First, when hypoxemia is present, because the compensatory response to metabolic alkalosis is hypoventilation, which can worsen the hypoxemia. Second, when pH is above 7.6, since alkalemia of this severity carries an increased risk of life-threatening cardiac arrhythmias and seizures.

Summary

Metabolic alkalosis is a disease process that increases plasma $[HCO_3^-]$, thereby producing alkalemia. Any marked increase in plasma $[HCO_3^-]$—aside from that arising as the compensation for respiratory acidosis—is by definition metabolic alkalosis. Because the kidneys, as part of their regulatory function, normally spill excess bicarbonate into the urine, metabolic alkalosis requires the presence of one or more "maintenance" factors. These factors raise the renal bicarbonate threshold, causing the kidney to retain excess bicarbonate, thus allowing plasma $[HCO_3^-]$ to rise. Key maintenance factors are volume depletion, chloride depletion, hypokalemia, and an elevated plasma aldosterone level. The most common clinical causes of metabolic alkalosis are: (1) loss of gastric fluid from vomiting or nasogastric drainage, (2) diuretics—either thiazide or loop—especially for the treatment of edema, (3) post-hypercapnic metabolic alkalosis, which can occur when a mechanically ventilated patient with compensated respiratory acidosis experiences an acute fall in PCO_2. These three causes produce metabolic alkalosis that can be treated with volume-expanding fluids (saline) and potassium; they are therefore called "volume-responsive." In contrast, "volume-resistant" metabolic alkalosis comprises a group of uncommon entities that do not respond to volume therapy. About 95 percent of metabolic alkalosis cases are due to volume-responsive causes. Only 5 percent of patients with metabolic alkalosis have volume-resistant causes.

Chapter 8

Respiratory Acidosis

In this chapter, we'll study respiratory acidosis in detail, focusing on its pathophysiology and clinical causes. We'll also briefly consider some important treatment concepts. As a reminder, respiratory acidosis is a disease process that increases arterial PCO_2, thereby producing acidemia. Any marked increase in plasma PCO_2—aside from that arising as the compensation for a metabolic alkalosis—is by definition respiratory acidosis.*

Respiratory acidosis has three main consequences. First, both acute and chronic hypercapnia (elevated PCO_2) cause cerebral vasodilation, which increases cranial blood flow and can raise intracranial pressure. Headache often results, especially at night, since baseline PCO_2 is normally higher during sleep. The increased perfusion (blood flow) can result in reddened eyes. Papilledema may occur if hypercapnia is severe. Second, acute hypercapnia can cause neurological, psychological, and neuromuscular effects. Mental acuity may decrease. Anxiety, disorientation, combativeness, hallucinations, delusions, delirium, or mania may appear. Muscle fasciculations may be present. If hypercapnia is severe, stupor or coma can develop. Third, when acidemia is severe, the sympathetic nervous system is strongly activated, so respiratory acidosis tends to produce tachycardia and hypertension. In patients breathing room air (i.e., no supplemental oxygen), hypercapnia is almost always accompanied by hypoxemia (low arterial PO_2), because respiratory defects severe enough to raise PCO_2 will also impair oxygen uptake. Therefore, it is not always clear whether a particular consequence is due to hypercapnia, hypoxemia, or both.

With that background, we're ready to learn how respiratory acidosis comes about.

Pathophysiology of Elevated PCO_2

Three main pathophysiological factors can elevate PCO_2 and thus cause respiratory acidosis: (1) neuromuscular chain defects, (2) pulmonary disease, and (3) increased CO_2 production. Whenever a particular disease, injury, or other clinical problem causes respiratory acidosis, one or more of these three factors is responsible. Let's look at these factors individually.

---

* **Terminology.** An elevated PCO_2 is termed hypercapnia. Therefore, respiratory acidosis is, by definition, simply hypercapnia that does not arise as compensation for metabolic alkalosis. The term respiratory acidosis is introduced and explained fully in Chapter 2. For a quick refresher, see the illustration on page 28. The concept of compensation is explained in Chapter 5.

1. Neuromuscular Chain Defects (a.k.a. Ventilatory Chain Defects)

Ventilation refers to the movement of air into and out of the lung. Normal ventilation requires an intact neuromuscular chain. The following figure shows the "links" in this chain:

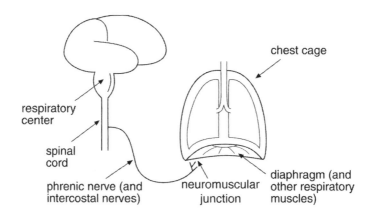

You can remember the links of this chain by tracing the sequence of normal inspiration. The **respiratory center** in the brainstem initiates the neural impulse. Since the brainstem is part of the central nervous system, this signal from the respiratory center is sometimes referred to as **central drive**. From the brain, the neural impulse travels down the cervical **spinal cord** and **phrenic nerves**, then across the **neuromuscular junction** (NMJ, the interface between nerve and muscle). The impulse stimulates the **diaphragm** and accessory respiratory muscles to contract. During this contraction, the diaphragm flattens and the **chest cage** expands.

Because these links are arranged in series (one after the other), normal inspiration requires that every link be intact. Like an actual chain, the ventilatory chain is only as strong as its weakest link. In fact, if the strength of several links is reduced, the impairment is cumulative. Regardless of which link or links are involved, any marked impairment in the chain reduces the overall ventilation of the lung. That is, total ventilation, a.k.a. minute ventilation, is reduced. This reduction may occur via a decrease in either depth of ventilation (tidal volume) or respiratory rate, or both. When total ventilation decreases, alveolar ventilation falls with it, causing arterial PCO_2 to rise. To summarize: neuromuscular chain defects reduce total ventilation, thereby reducing alveolar ventilation, which increases PCO_2 and causes hypercapnia.

2. Pulmonary Disease (a.k.a. Intrinsic Pulmonary Disease)

Unlike neuromuscular chain defects, which do not imply any damage to the lung itself, the terms "pulmonary disease" and "lung disease" refer specifically to defects in the lung. This fact is sometimes emphasized by saying "*intrinsic* pulmonary (or lung) disease." The adjective *intrinsic* emphasizes that the problem is actually *in* the lung. The following figure shows, in schematic form, the five major types of defects that occur in lung disease. Each image portrays an alveolus and the small airway (bronchiole) leading to it. Virtually all lung diseases comprise one or more of these five defects. Scan the figure, then keep reading:

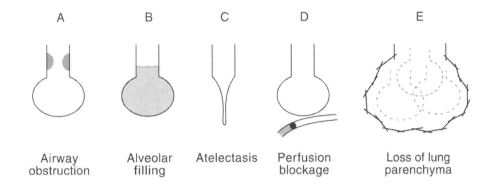

A	B	C	D	E
Airway obstruction	Alveolar filling	Atelectasis	Perfusion blockage	Loss of lung parenchyma

<u>Figure A</u> shows narrowing of a small airway that supplies an alveolus or group of alveoli. Narrowing can occur because of mucus blockage in the lumen, thickening of the airway wall (from acute swelling or chronic inflammation), or contraction of smooth muscle in the airway walls. Because airway narrowing reduces the amount of fresh air that reaches the affected alveoli, it can be thought of as causing localized hypoventilation. Airway narrowing is prominent in asthma and chronic bronchitis.

<u>Figure B</u> shows an alveolus filled with liquid or semi-liquid material. Air is entirely prevented from reaching the alveolar surface, so blood that perfuses this surface does not participate in gas exchange. The blood vessel therefore acts as a "shunt," effectively bypassing the lung and carrying venous blood directly into the systemic circulation without either picking up oxygen or unloading CO_2. Alveolar filling can be thought of as an extreme form of the localized hypoventilation seen in Figure A, in that ventilation in the affected alveoli falls to zero. Examples of alveolar filling are severe pulmonary edema, in which alveoli fill with fluid that has left the capillaries, and severe pneumonia, in which alveoli fill with pus.

<u>Figure C</u> shows the collapse of alveoli, a process termed atelectasis. If collapse is partial, ventilation in that region is reduced, similar to Figure A. If collapse is total, ventilation in that region is eliminated and the area acts as a shunt, as in Figure B.

<u>Figure D</u> shows blockage of a blood vessel, which reduces perfusion of part of the lung. Ventilation is normal but the loss of blood flow makes the alveoli completely ineffective as a gas exchange surface. In technical terms, the alveoli become "dead space" (in this context, "dead" means "unable to carry out gas exchange"). An example is pulmonary thromboembolism, which occurs when a blood clot, or thrombus, travels to the lung and lodges in a pulmonary artery.

<u>Figure E</u> shows the loss of alveolar walls and capillaries, as happens in emphysema. This wall loss greatly reduces the area of the lung's gas exchange surface, creating

abnormally large air spaces in the lung. (This process is analogous to knocking down the inside walls of a large apartment building, turning ordinary apartments into wide-open loft spaces and reducing the total surface area of walls in the building.)

These five defects are distinct in important ways but they share a crucial feature: all make the elimination of CO_2 by the lung less efficient. As a result, if PCO_2 is to remain at a normal level, total ventilation—the rate at which air moves into and out of the lung—must increase. These patients are said to have a higher **ventilatory requirement**, because a higher level of *ventilation* is *required* to maintain a normal PCO_2. If the patient cannot meet this higher ventilatory requirement—say, due to a neuromuscular chain defect, such as fatigue of the ventilatory muscles—PCO_2 will rise. In principle, a patient can meet a higher ventilatory requirement through a higher respiratory rate, greater tidal volume, or both.

In patients with intrinsic lung disease, total ventilation usually does increase somewhat, even if this increase is not sufficient to meet the new, higher ventilatory requirement. Several mechanisms are responsible for this increase in ventilation. First, lung disease directly stimulates sense receptors in the lung. These receptors are sensitive to bulk materials in the airspaces (fluid, mucus, pus, etc.), to vascular congestion, and to chemicals (e.g., inflammatory products from infected cells). Once stimulated, the receptors signal the respiratory center to increase central drive. Second, hypoxemia (low arterial PO_2), if present, further stimulates the respiratory center. Third, if hypercapnia is present, the high PCO_2 acts as a strong ventilatory stimulus. Any or all of these three mechanisms can cause the respiratory center to increase neural output to the ventilatory chain.

3. Increased Carbon Dioxide Production

A final influence on PCO_2 is the rate of CO_2 production by the tissues. If CO_2 production is increased, a greater rate of ventilation is needed to keep PCO_2 stable. That is, the ventilatory requirement rises. A patient with relatively healthy lungs and an intact ventilatory chain can easily increase ventilation. Think of how much your ventilation increases during physical exercise, which does not normally cause hypercapnia even though CO_2 production is markedly increased. However, patients with neuromuscular chain defects or intrinsic lung disease may not be able to increase ventilation sufficiently when CO_2 production rises. In these patients, elevated CO_2 production can contribute to, or even precipitate, hypercapnia.

Causes of high CO_2 production include fever (each $1°C$ rise of body temperature increases CO_2 production by about 13 percent), physical activity, anxiety, hyperthyroidism, and overfeeding with too many calories. Intrinsic lung disease also can raise CO_2 production. It can do this in two ways: increasing resistance to airflow and making lung tissue less compliant (stretchable). In either case, more muscular effort, which results in more CO_2 production, is required to carry out a given level of ventilation.

To summarize: when respiratory acidosis occurs, one or more of three pathophysiological processes is responsible: (1) ventilatory chain defect, (2) intrinsic pulmonary disease, and (3) increased CO_2 production. Let's now look at the actual diseases and other clinical problems that bring these pathophysiological processes into play.

Diseases that Cause Respiratory Acidosis

The diseases and other clinical problems that cause respiratory acidosis fall into two broad groups: those that involve intrinsic lung abnormalities (pulmonary causes) and those that do not (non-pulmonary causes). Let's consider these two categories separately, starting with non-pulmonary.

Non-Pulmonary Causes of Respiratory Acidosis

Most non-pulmonary causes of respiratory acidosis involve defects in the neuromuscular chain. Damage or impairment at any point in the chain can cause respiratory acidosis. You can divide the impairments into three categories: central drive, neural linkage, and respiratory muscles.

Central Drive

The most common cause of decreased central drive is overdose with drugs that suppress ventilation. Examples include opiates (e.g., heroin, morphine), barbiturates, and methaqualone (Quaalude). In patients with preexisting lung disease, even therapeutic levels of ventilatory suppressant medications can increase PCO_2. Post-surgical patients may have reduced ventilatory drive due to the residual effects of surgical anesthetics and paralytic agents; these patients are also at increased risk of airflow obstruction due to anesthesia-associated flaccidity of the soft palate; the risks are especially high in patients with a number of specific conditions, including sleep apnea, obesity-hypoventilation syndrome, and in patients undergoing bariatric surgery. Less common causes of depressed central drive include lesions of the respiratory center due to stroke, trauma, tumors, or infections.

Neural Linkage

Hypercapnia can be caused by trauma or diseases that affect the nerves that connect the respiratory center to the respiratory muscles. Examples include spinal cord damage above C5 (the phrenic nerves originate at C3–C5), damage to the phrenic nerves themselves, and disorders that affect neurotransmission, including: polio, amyotrophic lateral sclerosis (ALS, a.k.a. Lou Gehrig's Disease), multiple sclerosis, Guillain-Barre syndrome, botulism poisoning, myasthenia gravis, and aminoglycoside antibiotics (which can cause a myasthenia-like effect on neurotransmission).

Respiratory Muscles

Muscle weakness refers to a reduction of contractile force per given level of central drive. **Muscle fatigue** is a particular type of muscle weakness that is brought on by overwork and is relieved by muscle rest. Muscle weakness is sometimes severe enough to cause hypercapnia by itself, but even mild muscle weakness can hasten the onset of hypercapnia when other problems (e.g., intrinsic lung disease, defects of the chest wall) are present and increase the work of breathing. One common cause of muscle weakness is electrolyte depletion, especially low plasma levels of potassium, phosphate, or magnesium. By the time $[K^+]$ falls to about 2.5 mmol/l, or [phosphate] falls below about 1 mg/dl (0.3 mmol/l), severe muscle weakness may be present. Other important causes of muscle weakness are listed in the box near the end of this chapter (p. 113).

Pulmonary Causes of Respiratory Acidosis

Lung diseases, both acute and chronic, can cause respiratory acidosis. Common examples of *acute* lung disease include:

- pneumonia
- pulmonary edema
- pulmonary embolism
- acute asthmatic episode

Among the *chronic* lung diseases, the most common cause of hypercapnia is chronic obstructive pulmonary disease (COPD), which is most often caused by long-term cigarette smoking. COPD refers to two partly overlapping disease entities: emphysema and chronic bronchitis. Emphysema is characterized by extensive destruction of lung tissue. Chronic bronchitis is characterized by inflammation of the airways and excess mucus production. In general, hypercapnia, as well as hypoxemia, is most common among patients with chronic bronchitis, though even among these patients only some develop hypercapnia. In contrast, patients with a relatively pure emphysema pattern tend to maintain normal PO_2 and PCO_2 values. The reason for this difference is not known.

Respiratory Acidosis vs. Respiratory Alkalosis

The very same lung diseases that can produce respiratory acidosis (hypercapnia) can, in different circumstances, cause respiratory alkalosis (hypocapnia) instead. In fact, all of the acute lung diseases in the bulleted list above can produce either respiratory acidosis or alkalosis, depending on circumstances. It is important to understand what accounts for this variability, so let's consider that now.

Earlier in the chapter, I described how lung disease impairs CO_2 elimination and also can increase CO_2 production. Both these factors tend to *increase* PCO_2, causing respiratory acidosis. However, I also described how lung disease stimulates pulmonary sense receptors and, in addition, can produce systemic hypoxemia. Both these factors act to increase central drive, raising ventilation, and thus tend to *reduce* PCO_2, causing respiratory alkalosis. As you can see, lung disease brings into play factors that have opposing influences on PCO_2. Which of the opposing influences predominates—and hence whether the patient presents with respiratory acidosis or alkalosis—depends on two main variables: the *severity* of the lung disease and the *integrity* of the neuromuscular chain.

Patients with *mild* or *moderate* lung disease who also have a *fully functional* neuromuscular chain usually present with *hypo*capnia (low PCO_2). In these patients, the impairment of CO_2 excretion, and the increased rate of CO_2

production, are modest, and their effect on PCO_2 is outweighed by the effect of increased alveolar ventilation. The overall result of the lung disease is to decrease PCO_2. In contrast, patients with *severe* lung disease, or patients with any level of lung disease who also have an *impaired* neuromuscular chain (such as from muscle weakness or fatigue), tend to experience *hyper*capnia. In these patients, the impairment in CO_2 excretion and/or the increase in CO_2 production is marked, and these effects cannot be overcome by the limited increase in alveolar ventilation that the patient is able to muster. As a result, the overall effect of the lung disease is to increase PCO_2. To give an example: A patient with mild pneumonia and an intact neuromuscular chain will likely present with respiratory alkalosis; but if this pneumonia becomes more severe—especially if the respiratory muscles are fatigued from overwork—PCO_2 may rise and respiratory acidosis may develop.

Clinical Significance of Hypercapnia in Acute vs. Chronic Lung Disease

In patients with *acute* lung disease, respiratory acidosis is often an ominous sign. It may indicate that the patient is unstable and at risk of imminent respiratory collapse. In some patients, hypercapnia may signal the need for mechanical ventilation.

In contrast to these acutely ill patients, individuals with *chronic* hypercapnia from COPD may be relatively stable for long periods, even years. Due to the chronic nature of the condition, there is plenty of time for renal compensation to increase plasma $[HCO_3^-]$, so acidemia is mild. Some researchers have theorized that in COPD, hypercapnia may arise partly through a protective mechanism whereby ventilatory effort is automatically reduced to stave off muscle fatigue in the face of an elevated work load from the high airflow resistance.

Nonetheless, these chronically hypercapnic patients still remain in a somewhat precarious state. Any acute medical stress can rapidly increase PCO_2 to a higher (not-fully-compensated) level, causing more severe acidemia. Such acutely worsened patients are said to have "acute-on-chronic hypercapnia" or "acute-on-chronic ventilatory failure." Examples of stresses that can precipitate this acute rise in PCO_2 include: a superimposed lung infection, an acute episode of congestive heart failure with pulmonary edema, sedation with drugs that lower central drive, and sepsis.

Potassium Status in Respiratory Acidosis

Acute respiratory acidosis can slightly raise plasma $[K^+]$, though $[K^+]$ still usually remains within the normal range (often high-normal), unless other factors complicate the picture.* Chronic respiratory acidosis has no effect on plasma $[K^+]$.

---

*Mnemonic.** The rise in plasma $[K^+]$ is sometimes said to result from the exchange of K^+ and H^+ across the cell membrane, with H^+ entering cells and K^+ exiting into the ECF. This is not a bad way to remember the effect of acute respiratory acidosis on $[K^+]$. However, the actual mechanism is unknown.

Treatment Concepts

Hypercapnia can be understood in terms of the *load-strength model*. According to this model, hypercapnia arises when ventilatory *load* (the work required to carry out ventilation) exceeds neuromuscular *strength* (the output capacity of the neuro-muscular chain). This imbalance between load and strength is often multifactorial, the cumulative result of many small causes. Therefore, the treatment goal is to reduce load and increase strength at all possible points, as follows.

Reduce Ventilatory Load

Load can be broken down into four areas: upper airway, lung, "peri-lung," and CO_2 production:

1) *Upper airway.* Search for, and remove or treat, anything that could reduce air-flow in the nose, mouth, pharynx, and trachea. Consider swelling (even nasal allergies can contribute), food or other foreign objects including dentures, and blockages of the trachea or a bronchus.

2) *Lung.* Address all treatable intrinsic defects. Consider both definitive treatments (e.g., antibiotics, and diuretics and cardiac drugs for heart failure with pulmonary edema) and supportive or ongoing measures. Examples of the latter include postural drainage, chest physical therapy, hydration, low-salt diet, and weight loss. In patients with acute pulmonary edema, sitting the patient upright with legs hanging off the bed can reduce central blood volume and hence transiently improve the edema.

3) *"Peri-lung" (area around lung).* Consider factors that might physically hinder the flattening of the diaphragm, or the expansion of the chest cage, during inspiration. Consider and treat ascites, pleural effusion, pneumothorax, and respiratory "splinting" (self-immobilization) in response to the pain of trauma or surgery (treat pain while trying to minimize ventilatory suppression). In markedly obese patients, lying flat can cause the abdominal contents to push upwards on the bottom of the diaphragm, hindering inspiration. Sitting upright or tilting the bed into reverse Trendelenburg position (i.e., a flat bed surface with head higher than feet) may provide some relief. At home, this bed position can be obtained simply by putting blocks, bricks, or other sturdy bed-risers under the legs at the head of the bed.

4) *High CO_2 production.* An increase in CO_2 production raises the ventilatory re-quirement, and hence the work of breathing, since there is more CO_2 to eliminate. Treatable causes include fever, hyperthyroidism, physical activity, and over-feeding with too many calories.

Increase Neuromuscular Strength

Mentally trace the path of the neuromuscular chain (see illustration p. 106), ask-ing if any link could be impaired. Consider suppression of central drive from medications, neuromuscular disease, and a possible myasthenia-like reaction to aminoglycoside antibiotics. Consider and address all possible causes of muscle weakness. The following box lists important causes of muscle weakness:

Contributors to Muscle Weakness

Hypokalemia

Hypophosphatemia (low plasma phosphate)

Hypomagnesemia (low plasma magnesium)

Poor nutritional status

Sepsis

Acidemia

Hypoxemia

Anemia

Low cardiac output (impairs delivery of oxygen and nutrients
  to respiratory muscles)

Corticosteroid use

Hypothyroidism

Residual effects of muscle-paralyzing drugs used in surgery

Primary muscle disease (e.g., Duchenne muscular dystrophy)

Mechanical Ventilation (MV)

Deciding whether, and how, to implement MV by either endotracheal tube or non-invasive face-mask technologies is a complex topic beyond the scope of this book. But once the patient is on MV, a key point is that the clinician's role should *not* be one of passive waiting. Instead, the approach is the same as just described: the active and vigilant search for ways to decrease ventilatory load and increase neuromuscular strength. Muscle fatigue likely plays a role—and muscle rest on an *expertly managed* ventilator* may be necessary—but rest alone is usually insufficient. Identifying and treating factors that weaken the respiratory muscles (see box, above) may be necessary if the patient is to get off MV.

Summary

Respiratory acidosis is a disease process that increases arterial PCO_2, thereby producing acidemia. Any marked increase in plasma PCO_2—aside from the respiratory compensation for a metabolic alkalosis—is by definition respiratory acidosis. The ventilatory requirement, defined as the level of total ventilation needed to keep PCO_2 stable, rises with lung disease and with increased CO_2 production. If the work of breathing required to meet this higher ventilatory requirement cannot be maintained, PCO_2 rises. Clinical causes of hypercapnia are either

---

*__Clinical note__. Ensuring respiratory muscle rest in a mechanically ventilated patient requires specialized knowledge and can be technically difficult. Patients may actually be doing heavy work while ostensibly being "rested" on a ventilator. The most basic rule is to make sure the patient *looks* comfortable and does not appear to be straining, "bucking," or otherwise contracting respiratory muscles.

non-pulmonary or pulmonary. Non-pulmonary causes include a defect in any link of the neuromuscular chain. You can remember the links by mentally tracing the path of nerve impulses during inspiration: respiratory center → cervical spinal cord → phrenic nerve → neuromuscular junction → diaphragm (and other respiratory muscles). Pulmonary causes may be acute or chronic. Acute pulmonary disease often presents with hypocapnia (respiratory alkalosis), but PCO_2 may rise, thereby causing respiratory acidosis, if lung disease is severe or respiratory muscle weakness is present. Patients with hypercapnia from chronic lung disease (usually chronic bronchitis) are often relatively stable and well compensated. But these patients still remain in a somewhat precarious position because many acute stresses (e.g., lung infection, heart failure, sedative drugs, sepsis) can lead to an acute rise in PCO_2 ("acute-on-chronic hypercapnia"). Respiratory acidosis can be understood as occurring when ventilatory load exceeds neuromuscular strength. Treating respiratory acidosis involves addressing the multifactorial causes of this load-strength imbalance. Important causes of respiratory muscle weakness beyond simple fatigue are given in the box on page 113.

Chapter 9

Respiratory Alkalosis

In this chapter, we'll study respiratory alkalosis in detail, focusing on its patho-physiology and underlying clinical causes. We'll also briefly consider treatment. As a reminder, respiratory alkalosis is a disease process that decreases arterial PCO_2, thereby producing alkalemia. Any marked decline in plasma PCO_2—aside from that arising as the compensation for a metabolic acidosis—is by definition respiratory alkalosis. In other words: respiratory alkalosis is non-compensatory hypocapnia.*

Chronic respiratory alkalosis has few consequences, whereas *acute* respiratory alkalosis has many. First, acute respiratory alkalosis causes cerebral vasoconstriction, lowering intracranial blood flow and pressure. This relative ischemia can impair higher mental functioning and cause light-headedness and fainting. Second, acute respiratory alkalosis has neurologic effects, in particular peri-oral numbness, paresthesias (usually tingling) of fingers and toes, and carpopedal spasms (p. 5 footnote). Occasionally, generalized tetany, seizures, or coma can develop. Third, in persons who have coronary artery disease, but not usually in healthy persons, acute hypocapnia may increase the risk of cardiac arrhythmias. The neurologic and cardiac effects usually occur only at pH values of 7.55 or higher. In a patient with serious underlying disease, a pH of 7.55 is often poorly tolerated and may represent a medical emergency.

Let's now enter into the main part of this chapter by focusing on a key concept: that all respiratory alkalosis is caused by an abnormal elevation in central respiratory drive.

Respiratory Alkalosis is Caused by Elevated Central Drive

As discussed in Chapter 3, arterial PCO_2 is directly proportional to CO_2 production and inversely proportional to alveolar ventilation:

$$PCO_2 \propto CO_2 \text{ Production/Alveolar Ventilation}$$

In theory, then, respiratory alkalosis can result from either a fall in CO_2 production or a rise in alveolar ventilation. In a healthy person, ventilation slows to match any decrease in CO_2 production, thereby keeping PCO_2 constant. (Think of how

---

***Terminology.** A decreased PCO_2 is termed hyporcapnia. Therefore, respiratory alkalosis is, by definition, simply hypocapnia that does not arise as compensation for metabolic acidosis. The term respiratory alkalosis is introduced and explained in Chapter 2. For a quick refresher, see the illustration on page 28. The concept of compensation is explained in Chapter 5.

your breathing automatically slows when you sit quietly.) Therefore, as a practical matter, respiratory alkalosis is always caused by an abnormally high level of ventilation, one that is inappropriately elevated relative to the rate of CO_2 production.

This abnormally elevated ventilation occurs when some pathologic factor acts as a ventilatory stimulus. In contrast to respiratory acidosis, which can be caused by a defect anywhere along the neuromuscular chain (figure p. 106), respiratory alkalosis occurs only if (1) the entire neuromuscular chain is intact and (2) the respiratory center is pacing the chain to produce a high rate of ventilation. That is, *respiratory alkalosis is always caused by an increase in central drive.* Because elevated central drive is a key feature of respiratory alkalosis, it's useful to understand what factors elevate central drive clinically.

Pathophysiology: Abnormal Stimuli for Ventilation

Four pathophysiologic processes can cause an abnormal increase in central drive. Any time a disease or other clinical problem causes respiratory alkalosis, one or more of these four processes is responsible: (1) arterial hypoxemia or tissue hypoxia, (2) direct stimulation of pulmonary sense receptors by a disease process in the lung, (3) chemical or physical factors that directly affect the brain's medullary respiratory center, and (4) psychological factors. I already touched on the first two of these factors in the last chapter when discussing intrinsic lung disease, but here I'll say more.

1. Hypoxemia and Tissue Hypoxia

Arterial hypoxemia, defined as a low arterial PO_2, is sensed by chemosensors in the aortic arch and at the bifurcation of the carotid arteries. These sensors signal the medullary respiratory center, via nerve connections, to increase ventilatory drive. The increased ventilation homeostatically increases arterial PO_2 but, in the process, reduces PCO_2. Because of the shape of hemoglobin's saturation curve, most people have an adequate blood oxygen saturation (i.e., above 90 percent) any time PO_2 is above 60 mm Hg.* Once PO_2 falls below 60 mm Hg, hemoglobin saturation falls sharply and the hypoxemic drive to ventilation becomes increasingly strong. This drive is especially strong when hypoxemia is acute. Certain conditions cause tissue hypoxia (low tissue PO_2) even when arterial hypoxemia is not present. Examples include severe anemia, severe hypotension, and carbon monoxide poisoning. Like hypoxemia, tissue hypoxia can also increase ventilatory drive.

2. Stimulation of Pulmonary Sense Receptors

The walls of alveoli and conducting airways contain specialized sense receptors, including stretch receptors (mechanoreceptors) and irritant receptors (chemoreceptors). When stimulated by a pathologic process in the lung, these receptors increase their neural output to the medullary respiratory center, which can cause

---

*__Hint.__ The normal range for PO_2 is about 80–100 mm Hg, with younger people usually having PO_2 values in the high end of the range.

hyperventilation. For example, edema fluid in either the alveolar airspaces or lung interstitium can stimulate stretch receptors, and purulent debris from bacterial pneumonia can stimulate irritant receptors. These sense receptors can cause hyperventilation even if arterial PO_2 and oxygen delivery to tissues is normal.

3. Direct Stimulation of the Respiratory Center

Various toxins, chemicals, drugs, and physical insults to the medullary respiratory center can cause hyperventilation. These include normal physiologic factors (e.g., elevated progesterone during pregnancy), endogenous pathologic factors (e.g., un-detoxified waste products in liver disease), and drugs (e.g., salicylates). Sepsis, fever, and brain trauma also can stimulate ventilation.

4. Psychological Factors

Anxiety, stress, fear, and pain can all cause hyperventilation. Although this hyperventilation can sometimes be temporarily overridden by conscious effort, the pathways are largely involuntary.

To summarize: Respiratory alkalosis always indicates an increase of central drive. One or more of four pathophysiological processes is responsible for this increase: (1) hypoxemia or tissue hypoxia, (2) stimulation of pulmonary sense receptors, (3) direct stimulation of the medullary respiratory center, (4) psychologic factors. Let's now look at the actual diseases and other clinical problems that bring these four pathophysiological processes into play.

Diseases that Cause Respiratory Alkalosis

The diseases and other clinical problems that cause respiratory alkalosis fall into two groups: those that involve intrinsic lung abnormalities (pulmonary causes) and those that do not (non-pulmonary causes). These are the same two categories we distinguished for respiratory acidosis. Let's consider pulmonary diseases first.

Pulmonary Causes of Respiratory Alkalosis

Most kinds of lung disease can cause respiratory alkalosis. Examples include:

- pneumonia
- pulmonary embolism
- interstitial fibrosis
- asthma
- pulmonary edema

In each of these diseases, one or more of the above four hyperventilation-causing factors is involved. For example, in bacterial pneumonia, all of the following may stimulate ventilation: hypoxemia with tissue hypoxia, stimulation of both stretch and irritant receptors in the lung, fever, and anxiety. As I mentioned in Chapter 8 (pp. 110–111), if the underlying lung disease worsens, or if respiratory muscle fatigue sets in, PCO_2 can increase and respiratory acidosis can supervene.

Non-Pulmonary Causes of Respiratory Alkalosis

As with the pulmonary causes, the non-pulmonary causes stimulate hyperventilation by one of the four pathophysiological mechanisms described above. Some important examples follow.

Sepsis

Sepsis, septic syndrome, and septicemia all refer to the presence in the blood of pathogenic microorganisms, or of toxic products associated with the organisms, leading to systemic (i.e., body-wide) clinical manifestations. Hyperventilation with respiratory alkalosis is common in these patients. Causes include gram-negative, gram-positive, and fungal organisms. Several mechanisms can mediate the hyperventilation, including stimulation of chemoreceptors in the respiratory center by cytokines or other toxic byproducts of the microorganisms.

Liver Disease

Respiratory alkalosis can develop with all types of chronic liver disease. With severe disease, PCO_2 may fall to below 30 mm Hg. The cause of the hyperventilation is uncertain but may involve increases in plasma progesterone, estradiol, and the nitrogenous wastes that are usually broken down by the liver. Liver disease may also cause physiological (normally present) shunt vessels in the lung to dilate and thus carry more blood. These vessels bypass the alveolar capillary beds, shunting unoxygenated blood from the pulmonary artery directly into the pulmonary vein. This can result in hypoxemia, further stimulating hyperventilation. Though the mechanism is not known, the dilation of these shunt vessels may be pathophysiologically related to the dilation of small blood vessels in skin that cause "spider nevi" in patients with liver disease.

Salicylate Intoxication

Salicylate intoxication can cause both respiratory alkalosis and metabolic acidosis, as discussed in Chapter 6 (p. 75).

Brain Lesions

Injury or inflammation of the brain can cause either hyper- or hypoventilation. Midbrain lesions (especially strokes) can cause *central hyperventilation*, which is characterized by constant, rapid, deep breathing. Diffuse injuries (often secondary to trauma, hemorrhage, or chronic hypoxia) can cause *Cheyne-Stokes respiration* (pronounced "chain-stokes," sometimes called periodic respiration), which is characterized by alternating periods of hyperventilation and apnea (cessation of ventilation).

Cyanotic heart disease

Any cardiac disorder that causes right-to-left shunting within the heart can cause hypoxemia and thereby stimulate hyperventilation. In right-to-left shunting, unoxygenated blood (right heart) pours into a cardiac chamber that normally contains oxygenated blood (left heart). Examples include septal defects and patent ductus arteriosus with reversal of flow.

Pregnancy

Respiratory alkalosis is a normal part of pregnancy and is not pathologic. Stimulation of the respiratory center by progesterone is the likely cause. Hyperventilation begins early in pregnancy and usually remains stable or increases somewhat as pregnancy progresses. Often, PCO_2 falls to around 30 mm Hg and renal compensation reduces arterial $[HCO_3^-]$ to around 20 mmol/l, with a fair amount of variation among individuals. Plasma pH is often high normal. The hyperventilation of pregnancy is often associated with dyspnea (a subjective sense of shortness of breath) on light exertion or even at rest.

High Altitude

Because the partial pressure of atmospheric oxygen decreases with altitude, high altitude reduces arterial PO_2 and can thus result in hyperventilation and respiratory alkalosis. This effect usually starts at some point above 5,000 feet.

Psychogenic Hyperventilation

Some people hyperventilate in response to psychologic stimuli such as anxiety, stress, fear, anger, or pain. This process is referred to by various names, including psychogenic hyperventilation, primary hyperventilation, and anxiety-hyperventilation syndrome. In these individuals, the abnormal sensations produced by the hypocapnia and alkalemia can add to the underlying anxiety, contributing to a vicious cycle of continued hyperventilation. Some patients present with a purely acute episode. Others experience a degree of chronic hyperventilation (with $[HCO_3^-]$ slightly decreased, as compensation) and then become symptomatic if the hyperventilation intensifies. In some patients, acute episodes may present as panic attacks.

Potassium Status in Respiratory Alkalosis

Acute respiratory alkalosis can slightly lower plasma $[K^+]$, though $[K^+]$ usually remains within the normal range (often low normal) unless other hypokalemia-causing factors are also present. The mechanism is not known. Chronic respiratory alkalosis has no effect on plasma $[K^+]$.

Treatment Concepts

Except when respiratory alkalosis is acute and severe, and thus associated with a very high pH, hypocapnia is not itself dangerous and no attempt is usually made to directly increase PCO_2. The major importance of respiratory alkalosis is that it can alert you to the presence of an underlying disease. Because this underlying disease may be acutely life threatening (e.g., sepsis), it is crucial to search for and identify the underlying cause without delay. A related point is that if you have already identified a condition that can potentially causes respiratory alkalosis, it is often *not* necessary to determine with certainty (i.e., by blood gas) whether respiratory alkalosis is actually present. For example, if you diagnose mild asthma in a clinically stable patient, you can reasonably suspect that a mild respiratory alkalosis exists—but there is often no need to verify this fact since the alkalosis itself needs no treatment and you already know what the underlying condition is. (However, there may be other reasons to get a blood gas in a patient with suspected respiratory alkalosis, such as definitively ruling out hypoxemia, ruling out additional suspected acid-base disturbances, or getting a baseline PCO_2 in a patient you think may deteriorate.) Finally, it is important to remember that hyperventilation may indicate either respiratory alkalosis or compensation for metabolic acidosis. Therefore, if you detect hyperventilation clinically, you should always consider the possibility that metabolic acidosis may be the primary disorder.

Summary

Respiratory alkalosis is a disease process that decreases arterial PCO_2, thereby producing alkalemia. Any marked decline in plasma PCO_2—aside from the compensation for a metabolic acidosis—is by definition respiratory alkalosis. Respiratory alkalosis is caused by an abnormal ventilatory stimulus, usually one or more of the following: (1) hypoxemia or tissue hypoxia, (2) stimulation of lung sense receptors by pulmonary disease, (3) chemical or physical factors that directly affect the medullary respiratory center, and (4) psychologic factors such as pain, fear, or anxiety. Clinical causes are pulmonary and non-pulmonary. Pulmonary causes include most of the common lung diseases (e.g., asthma, pneumonia, pulmonary embolism, pulmonary edema, interstitial fibrosis). These diseases most often present with respiratory alkalosis, but PCO_2 can rise, leading to respiratory acidosis, if the disease is very severe or associated with respiratory muscle fatigue. Non-pulmonary causes include sepsis, liver disease, salicylate intoxication, brain lesions, cyanotic heart disease, normal pregnancy, and psychogenic hyperventilation. The major clinical importance of respiratory alkalosis is that it can alert you to the presence of a potentially life-threatening underlying disease (e.g., sepsis), which should be sought and identified rapidly.

Chapter 10

Mixed Disturbances

In this brief chapter, you'll study some common clinical scenarios that cause mixed (a.k.a. complex) acid-base disturbances. Becoming familiar with these scenarios will help you recognize mixed disturbances when you see them. As a reminder, the term mixed disturbance refers to the simultaneous presence of two or more primary acid-base disturbances in the same patient. For example, a patient who has both metabolic acidosis and respiratory alkalosis is said to have a mixed disturbance. The material presented here builds on Chapters 6–9, so I'm going to presume you already know the pathophysiology of the individual primary disturbances that together make up the mixed disturbances. (You can refer back to Chapters 6–9 if you need a refresher at any point.) For first-time students of acid-base, read for meaning but don't worry about memorizing; then revisit and review the chapter as your clinical experience grows. To keep things short and simple, I present this chapter in the form of an alphabetical list.

Alcoholic Ketoacidosis (AKA)

Following a sustained drinking-vomiting binge, metabolic acidosis from AKA may co-exist with metabolic alkalosis from vomiting. Plasma $[HCO_3^-]$ may be high, low, or normal, depending whether the metabolic acidosis or alkalosis predominates. Respiratory alkalosis may also exist, whether or not metabolic alkalosis is present, as a result of chronic liver disease from alcoholism, aspiration pneumonia, or alcohol withdrawal.

Arteriopuncture

Yes, you read correctly. The arteriopuncture that is required for an ABG can sometimes be frightening and painful enough to cause the patient to hyperventilate, resulting in a PCO_2 that is lower than it would be otherwise. This arteriopuncture-related reduction in PCO_2 can occur whether the patient's initial PCO_2 is normal, high, or low. Thus, it can potentially affect the PCO_2 of virtually any blood gas. For example, it can cause a simple disturbance (say, a simple metabolic acidosis) to produce a blood gas that looks mixed (a mixed metabolic acidosis and respiratory alkalosis). Although I am not aware of any studies about this, it is usually assumed that this phenomenon is only occasionally pronounced enough to cause a clinically meaningful change in PCO_2. Therefore, in most situations it's best to simply interpret the blood gas at face value, without wondering whether an arteriopuncture-related reduction in PCO_2 has occurred. Still, you should keep the possibility in the back of your mind, particularly when arteriopuncture is unusually difficult or painful, or when the patient is very anxious about the arteriopuncture.

Asthma

An asthmatic episode can present with respiratory alkalosis or, when severe, respiratory acidosis. Among the most seriously ill of these patients, if severe hypoxemia is present, lactic acidosis may develop.*

Cardiac Arrest

Cardiac arrest (standstill) always causes at least some lactic acidosis because of low tissue perfusion. Cardiac arrest is normally accompanied by ventilatory arrest, resulting in respiratory acidosis (which may persist if artificial ventilation is inadequate).**

COPD Patients Treated with Diuretics, Theophylline, or Steroids

These medications, which are commonly prescribed for COPD patients, all can cause metabolic alkalosis. If hypercapnia is present from the COPD, the metabolic alkalosis creates a mixed disturbance, so $[HCO_3^-]$ is higher than its predicted compensated level. Diuretics are used to treat peripheral edema, which may result from the cor pulmonale that sometimes develops in COPD patients. Theophylline, used to reduce airflow resistance in the lung, can cause vomiting. Glucocorticoid steroids, used to reduce pulmonary inflammation, have some mineralocorticoid (aldosterone-like) actions, which can both generate and maintain metabolic alkalosis (pp. 93–94).

COPD Patients with an Acute Respiratory Disturbance

COPD patients with stable, compensated hypercapnia may experience acute changes in PCO_2 due to acute respiratory acidosis or alkalosis. Most common is an acute rise in PCO_2 ("acute-on-chronic respiratory acidosis") due to an acute lung infection.

Diarrhea (severe)

Diarrhea usually causes a simple metabolic acidosis. However, if diarrhea is severe and sustained (e.g., in cholera), ECF and plasma volume may be so reduced that tissue hypoperfusion results, causing a superimposed lactic acidosis. Thus, two different causes of metabolic acidosis are present.***

---

*__Clinical note.__ An even more frequent cause of elevated plasma lactate may be the beta-adrenergic medications (e.g., albuterol) that are often used to treat asthma. It appears that these medications themselves sometimes raise plasma lactate levels as a side effect. This hyperlactatemia may occur with or without causing a noticeable reduction in plasma $[HCO_3^-]$.

**__Going further.__ Even if ventilation is adequate, reduced blood circulation can cause PCO_2 *inside cells* to rise ("intracellular respiratory acidosis"). With reduced tissue perfusion, CO_2 leaving tissues enters a smaller volume of blood, raising capillary blood PCO_2. This high capillary PCO_2 decreases the diffusion gradient from tissue to blood, so tissue PCO_2 rises as well. In this situation, arterial PCO_2 is normal if ventilation is adequate, since the lung still clears excess CO_2 from whatever blood passes through it. In contrast, mixed venous blood PCO_2 may be elevated.

***__Terminology.__ Although mixed disturbances usually take the form of two different primary disorders (e.g., metabolic acidosis + respiratory alkalosis), the definition of the term mixed disturbance also allows for two different causes of the same primary disorder (e.g., metabolic acidosis + metabolic acidosis), as in this case.

Liver Disease

Liver disease commonly presents with respiratory alkalosis. When liver disease is severe, several mixed disturbances are possible. The most common is respiratory alkalosis plus a metabolic alkalosis from either (a) diuretics given for ascites or (b) vomiting associated with nausea from the disease.

Pregnancy with Vomiting

Pregnancy itself usually causes a compensated respiratory alkalosis. If nausea and vomiting occur, a superimposed metabolic alkalosis can develop. The respiratory and metabolic alkaloses both increase pH, so alkalemia may be prominent even if the component disorders are mild.

Pulmonary Edema

Pulmonary edema can cause either respiratory alkalosis or respiratory acidosis. When pulmonary edema is due to failure of the left ventricle (cardiogenic pulmonary edema), a superimposed lactic acidosis can develop secondary to tissue hypoperfusion.

Salicylates

Salicylate overdose can cause both metabolic acidosis and respiratory alkalosis, as discussed in Chapter 6 (p. 75)

Septic Shock

Septic shock often presents with respiratory alkalosis due to stimulation of the respiratory center. Lactic acidosis, secondary to tissue hypoperfusion, sometimes also occurs.

Chapter 11

Diagnosis with Arterial Blood Gases

In the world of clinical acid-base, there are several laboratory tests that are so important that we can think of them as the quintessential acid-base tests. These tests deserve full and detailed explanations accompanied by multiple practice problems. In this chapter, we'll study the best known of these tests: the arterial blood gas.*

The term **Arterial blood gas (ABG)** refers to a specific set of tests done on an arterial blood sample. The ABG gives four key pieces of information: pH, PCO_2, $[HCO_3^-]$, and PO_2. The name *blood gas* is really a partial misnomer, since H^+ and bicarbonate are not gases. Because PO_2 it is not directly relevant to acid-base diagnosis (you don't need to know PO_2 to diagnose the four primary disturbances) we'll focus on pH, PCO_2, and $[HCO_3^-]$. These are sometimes called the three acid-base variables. In most labs, the normal arterial values (and normal ranges) are:

pH	=	7.40 (7.35–7.45)
PCO_2	=	40 (35–45)
$[HCO_3^-]$	=	24 (21–27)

How are these values measured? Blood is drawn from an artery, and a blood gas machine (analyzer) directly measures pH and PCO_2. The $[HCO_3^-]$, however, is not measured. Instead, the lab *calculates* this value by plugging the values for pH and PCO_2 into a mathematical formula (a rearranged version of the Henderson-Hasselbalch equation). Most blood gas analyzers do this calculation automatically. Because $[HCO_3^-]$ is not measured directly, it is sometimes mistakenly thought to be inaccurate. In fact, the calculated value is quite accurate.

Puncturing an artery to get a blood sample is relatively invasive; it is painful and carries a small but real risk of serious complications.** For this reason, you will not

---

* **Hint.** If you jumped directly to this chapter for a focused tutorial on blood gas interpretation, I recommend that you read Chapter 5 ("Compensation") first. Think of Chapter 5 as Part 1, and this chapter as Part 2, of the tutorial.

** **Clinical note.** Blood is usually drawn from the radial artery, occasionally from the femoral artery (usually in an emergency), and sometimes, especially in the ICU, via an indwelling arterial catheter ("arterial line"). When blood is obtained via puncture of the radial artery, the Allen test must be performed first, to ensure that the ulnar artery and other collateral vessels supplying the hand are patent and functioning.

get a blood gas for all patients. There are few absolute rules for when a blood gas is needed, but many clinicians consider a blood gas important when you suspect one of the following:

- A significant acute respiratory illness

- A significant acute exacerbation of a chronic respiratory illness (such as an acute respiratory infection in a patient with COPD)

- A chronic respiratory illness for which you lack a reliable baseline ABG

- A severe or rapidly progressive acid-base disorder of any type, whether respiratory or metabolic

- A mixed disturbance in which the component disturbances are clinically significant.

Interpreting the Blood Gas: A Three-Step Method

We're now going to learn blood-gas interpretation systematically, using a three-step method. In a moment, we'll study the steps in detail, but this box gives you a preview. Take a moment to study it.

Step 1: Assess the pH. Acidemia indicates acidosis. Alkalemia indicates alkalosis.

Step 2: Determine whether the "-osis" is metabolic (defined as a primary change in $[HCO_3^-]$) or respiratory (defined as a primary change in PCO_2).

Step 3: Use the rules of thumb to see if compensation is in the expected range.

In this part of the chapter, we'll focus just on Steps 1 and 2. These are the foundational steps and it's useful to master them first. Afterwards, we'll add Step 3.

STEP 1. Look at the pH. If acidemia (low pH) is present, there must be an acidosis. If alkalemia (high pH) is present, there must be an alkalosis. There is no other way for acidemia or alkalemia to arise. An "-emia" always implies the corresponding "-osis."

STEP 2. Determine whether the "-osis" is metabolic or respiratory, as follows: If the patient has acidosis, proceed according to *a*. If the patient has alkalosis, proceed according to *b*:

a. *Acidosis.* If $[HCO_3^-]$ is low, metabolic acidosis is present. If PCO_2 is high, respiratory acidosis is present. If $[HCO_3^-]$ is low *and* PCO_2 is high, both metabolic acidosis and respiratory acidosis are present (i.e., there is a mixed disturbance).

b. *Alkalosis.* If [HCO$_3^-$] is high, metabolic alkalosis is present. If PCO$_2$ is low, respiratory alkalosis is present. If [HCO$_3^-$] is high *and* PCO$_2$ is low, both metabolic alkalosis and respiratory alkalosis are present (i.e., there is a mixed disturbance).

The following flow chart shows Steps 1 and 2 visually. I've incorporated normal values for pH, [HCO$_3^-$], and PCO$_2$ into the figure. Make sure you understand the logic behind each step:

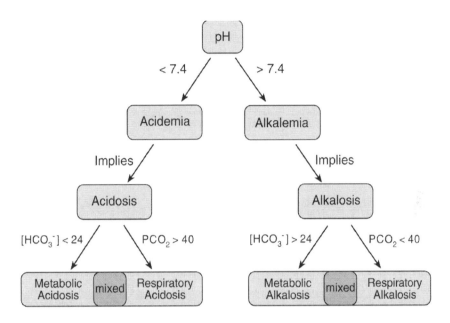

Note: [HCO$_3^-$] in mmol/l, PCO$_2$ in mm Hg

Practicing Steps 1 & 2

Steps 1 and 2 form the heart of ABG diagnosis, so it's useful to pause for practice before moving to Step 3. Try to interpret each of the five ABGs below. Refer to the above text and flow chart as needed. Work each problem as fully as you can, then check your answer and thought process against the solution.

Patient 1.   pH = 7.30   [HCO$_3^-$] = 14   PCO$_2$ = 30

Solution. Step 1: A pH of 7.30 is acidemia, so you know an acidosis is present. Step 2: To see if this acidosis is metabolic or respiratory, look at both [HCO$_3^-$] and PCO$_2$. It doesn't matter which you start with. I'll begin with [HCO$_3^-$]. The low [HCO$_3^-$] indicates metabolic acidosis. In other words, the [HCO$_3^-$] can account for a low pH, so you know that metabolic acidosis is definitely present. Now look at PCO$_2$. It is low. A low PCO$_2$ does not represent an acidosis. It cannot by itself account for a low pH. In fact, if [HCO$_3^-$] were normal, a low

PCO$_2$ would cause alkalemia, not acidemia. You therefore know that the decrease in PCO$_2$ is not the cause of the acidemia but, rather, is the result of respiratory compensation, which follows the same-direction rule. That is, the compensatory variable (PCO$_2$) moved in the same "direction"—low—as [HCO$_3^-$]. <u>Diagnosis</u>: metabolic acidosis.

Patient 2. pH = 7.57 [HCO$_3^-$] = 42 PCO$_2$ = 47

Solution. Step 1: A pH of 7.57 is alkalemia, so an alkalosis is present. Step 2: To determine whether this alkalosis is metabolic or respiratory, look at both [HCO$_3^-$] and PCO$_2$. It doesn't matter which you start with. I'll start with [HCO$_3^-$]. The high [HCO$_3^-$] indicates metabolic alkalosis. In other words, the [HCO$_3^-$] can account for a high pH, so you know a metabolic alkalosis is definitely present. PCO$_2$ is also high. A high PCO$_2$ is not an alkalosis. It cannot account for a high pH. In fact, if [HCO$_3^-$] were normal, a high PCO$_2$ would cause acidemia, not alkalemia. You therefore know that the rise in PCO$_2$ is not causing the alkalemia but rather is the result of respiratory compensation, which follows the same-direction rule. That is, the compensatory variable (PCO$_2$) moved in the same direction—high—as the [HCO$_3^-$]. <u>Diagnosis</u>: metabolic alkalosis.

Patient 3. pH = 7.57 [HCO$_3^-$] = 18 PCO$_2$ = 18

Solution. Step 1: A pH of 7.57 is alkalemia, so alkalosis is present. Step 2: To determine whether this alkalosis is metabolic or respiratory, look at both [HCO$_3^-$] and PCO$_2$. I'll start with [HCO$_3^-$]. A low [HCO$_3^-$] is not an alkalosis. It cannot account for the alkalemia. In fact, a low [HCO$_3^-$] by itself is a metabolic acidosis and causes acidemia. Therefore, [HCO$_3^-$] must be low because it is compensating for a low PCO$_2$ (respiratory alkalosis), according to the same-direction rule. So, even before you look at PCO$_2$, you can infer that it will be low. Turning to PCO$_2$, you see that PCO$_2$ is in fact low. A low PCO$_2$ is an alkalosis and can account for a high pH. <u>Diagnosis</u>: respiratory alkalosis.

Patient 4. pH = 7.60 [HCO$_3^-$] = 32 PCO$_2$ = 34

Solution. Step 1: A pH of 7.60 is alkalemia, so an alkalosis is present. Step 2: The high [HCO$_3^-$] can account for a high pH. That is, a high [HCO$_3^-$] causes alkalemia. Therefore, a metabolic alkalosis is present. Turning to PCO$_2$, you see that it is low. A low PCO$_2$ *also* can account for a high pH. That is, a low PCO$_2$ increases pH. Therefore, a respiratory alkalosis is also present. So [HCO$_3^-$] and PCO$_2$ can each independently account for the direction of the pH change. Put differently, both the metabolic and respiratory components are pushing pH in the same direction. Therefore, both metabolic alkalosis and respiratory alkalosis are present. By definition, this is a mixed disturbance: more than one primary disturbance occurring simultaneously in the same patient. Notice that the individual disturbances are not severe yet the pH is very abnormal. This is what you expect when two separate disturbances push pH in the same direction. <u>Diagnosis</u>: mixed metabolic alkalosis and respiratory alkalosis.

Patient 5. pH = 7.39   [HCO_3^-] = 22 PCO_2 = 38

Solution. This is a normal blood gas. pH, [HCO_3^-] and PCO_2 are all within their normal arterial ranges (pH 7.35–7.45, [HCO_3^-] 21–27, PCO_2 35–45). Some mixed disturbances can present with a normal blood gas, so you are not absolutely ruling out an acid-base disturbance. For example, if metabolic acidosis (say, from diarrhea) occurs with an equal-strength metabolic alkalosis (say, from vomiting), there will be offsetting effects on [HCO_3^-], and a normal blood gas will result. But the blood gas itself is completely normal and does not point to any problems. Any hint of a mixed disturbance, if there is one, will have to come from the history, physical exam, or other tests. <u>Diagnosis</u>: normal blood gas.

Step 3: Assessing the Level of Compensation

In a simple acid-base disturbance, one (not both) of the two key "-osis" variables ([HCO_3^-] or PCO_2) will account for the direction of the pH deviation. Assuming enough time has passed for compensation to develop, the variable that cannot account for the pH change will be deviated in a manner consistent with the "same-direction rule." For example, if pH is low and PCO_2 is *elevated* (respiratory acidosis), [HCO_3^-] will also be *elevated* (compensation). However—and this is a key point—it is possible that the compensatory variable moved in the right *direction* (consistent with the same-direction rule) but not to the appropriate *degree*. Put differently, within the broad prediction provided by the same-direction rule, you may find either over-compensation (the compensatory variable moved too far from its baseline) or under-compensation (the compensatory variable did not move far enough from its baseline). In either of these situations, a likely explanation is that an additional acid-base disturbance is affecting the compensatory variable, causing it to be either too high or too low.

To detect this kind of subtle, additional disturbance, you must proceed to Step 3. This step involves using "rules of thumb" to check if compensation is in the expected numerical range. The rules of thumb were introduced in Chapter 5 and are summarized in the table below. If the actual level of the compensatory variable does not match the value predicted by the rule, an additional disturbance may be present.

Scan the table on the following page, then keep reading.

Compensatory Rules of Thumb		
Disorder & Primary Change	**Compensation**	**Rule of Thumb**
Metabolic acidosis $\downarrow [HCO_3^-]$	$\downarrow PCO_2$	$PCO_2 = (1.5 \times [HCO_3^-]) + 8, \pm 2$ "Winters' formula"
Metabolic alkalosis $\uparrow [HCO_3^-]$	$\uparrow PCO_2$	PCO_2 increases 0.7 mm Hg for each 1 mmol/l increase in $[HCO_3^-]$, ± 5 mm Hg "The 0.7 Rule."
Respiratory acidosis $\uparrow PCO_2$	$\uparrow [HCO_3^-]$	<u>Acute:</u> For each 10 mm Hg increase in PCO_2, $[HCO_3^-]$ increases 1 mmol/l <u>Chronic:</u> For each 10 mm Hg increase in PCO_2, $[HCO_3^-]$ increases 3.5 – 5.0 mmol/l
Respiratory alkalosis $\downarrow PCO_2$	$\downarrow [HCO_3^-]$	<u>Acute:</u> For each 10 mm Hg decrease in PCO_2, $[HCO_3^-]$ decreases 2 mmol/l <u>Chronic:</u> For each 10 mm Hg decrease in PCO_2, $[HCO_3^-]$ decreases 4 mmol/l

Notes

1. **General**. Other rules of thumb exist. Most rules are reasonably accurate and none are perfect, including those given here. If you encounter a well-accepted rule that you like better or can remember more easily, use it.

2. **Metabolic alkalosis.** The compensatory response to metabolic alkalosis is hypoventilation, which lowers PO_2 as it raises PCO_2. Because hypoxemia stimulates ventilation, it is unusual to see a compensatory PCO_2 above 55 mm Hg.

3. **Respiratory acidosis.** The 3.5–5.0 range presumes that simple chronic respiratory acidosis can present with a normal pH. Controversy surrounding this issue is discussed on page 56. If you prefer to assume that chronic respiratory acidosis always presents with acidemia, use the single value of 3.5 instead of the 3.5–5.0 range.

These compensatory rules assume that enough time has passed for compensation to develop fully. This assumption is usually valid for *metabolic* disturbances (metabolic acidosis and metabolic alkalosis) because most of these develop fairly gradually, letting compensation—which takes just 12–24 hours to complete— build along with the disturbance. However, if the disturbance has a rapid onset (lactic acidosis is an example), there may be a lag between the onset of the disturbance and the appearance of compensation. Therefore, when compensation for a metabolic acidosis or alkalosis is less complete than the rule predicts, you should at least *consider* the possibility that compensation will develop more fully with time.

The situation is somewhat different for *respiratory* disturbances. Since compensation for respiratory disturbances takes longer to complete (3–5 days), you will often encounter patients who are not yet compensated. Therefore, separate rules of thumb are used for acute and chronic respiratory disturbances. If the patient just developed the disturbance, you'll use the acute rule. If the patient developed the disturbance more than 3–5 days ago, you'll use the chronic rule. If the patient developed the disturbance within the window between the acute and chronic time frames (say, between 1 and 3 days ago), $[HCO_3^-]$ should be between the levels predicted by the acute and chronic rules.

Practicing Steps 1–3 Together

The rest of this chapter consists of mini-cases with solutions. Here you'll work all three steps. I'll start with straightforward problems and then introduce a few complexities. As before, work each problem as fully as you can before checking the solution. As a training exercise, you may find it helpful to work the problems in writing, sketching out the steps, your thought process, and calculations. For easy reference, here are the three steps again. I'll state them using slightly different words from before, but the steps are the same:

Interpreting the Blood Gas in Three Steps

Step 1: Assess pH. Acidemia implies acidosis. Alkalemia implies alkalosis.

Step 2: Determine whether the "-osis" is metabolic or respiratory by seeing which variable ($[HCO_3^-]$ or PCO_2) can account for the direction of the pH change.

Step 3: Use the rules of thumb to see if compensation is as predicted.

Patient 6. A woman with a history of severe bulimia has this blood gas:

$$pH = 7.51 \quad [HCO_3^-] = 38 \quad PCO_2 = 49$$

Solution. Steps 1 & 2 tell you that the patient has metabolic alkalosis—consistent with the history (since vomiting can cause metabolic alkalosis). For Step 3, use the metabolic alkalosis rule of thumb. Since you don't know the patient's actual baseline values for $[HCO_3^-]$ and PCO_2, use the classic (mid-point of normal range) values of 24 and 40, respectively, as your assumed starting points. $[HCO_3^-]$ is 14 mmol/l above normal (38 − 24 = 14). According to the rule, multiply 14 × 0.7, which gives you 9.8. Round this 9.8 to 10. Adding 10 to the starting PCO_2 (40) gives a predicted PCO_2 of 50. Building in the ±5 gives a predicted range of range of 45–55 (50 − 5 = 45, 50 + 5 = 55). PCO_2 is well within this range, suggesting that compensation is appropriate. <u>Diagnosis</u>: simple metabolic alkalosis.

Patient 7. A man with poorly controlled insulin-dependent diabetes:

$$pH = 7.22 \qquad [HCO_3^-] = 8 \qquad PCO_2 = 22$$

Solution. Steps 1 & 2 indicate metabolic acidosis—consistent with the history (diabetic ketoacidosis). For Step 3, use the Winters' formula:

$$
\begin{aligned}
\text{Predicted } PCO_2 \ = \ & (1.5 \times [HCO_3^-]) + 8, \pm 2 \\
& (1.5 \times 8) + 8, \pm 2 \\
& 12 + 8, \pm 2 \\
& 20 \pm 2 \\
& 20 + 2 = 22 \\
& 20 - 2 = 18 \\
& 18 - 22 \text{ mm Hg}
\end{aligned}
$$

Compensation is in the expected range of 18–22. <u>Diagnosis</u>: simple metabolic acidosis.

Patient 8. A toddler aspirated a marble two hours ago and is in respiratory distress:

$$pH = 7.26 \qquad [HCO_3^-] = 28 \qquad PCO_2 = 60$$

Solution. Steps 1 & 2 point to respiratory acidosis. The history and physical exam suggest the acidosis is acute, so use the acute rule of thumb for Step 3. According to the rule, each 10 mm Hg rise in PCO_2 results in a 1 mmol/l rise in $[HCO_3^-]$. Since PCO_2 is elevated by 20 from an assumed baseline of 40 (60 – 40 = 20), $[HCO_3^-]$ should be about 2 mmol/l above its starting point. One way to approach the numbers is to work backwards, subtracting this 2 mmol/l from the observed $[HCO_3^-]$ of 28. This gives an assumed starting $[HCO_3^-]$ of 26, which is within the normal arterial $[HCO_3^-]$ range of 21–27. So the picture fits together: an acute rise of PCO_2 from 40 to 60 causing an acute rise in $[HCO_3^-]$ from 26 to 28. The history and physical exam are consistent with the laboratory findings. Had the history and/or physical exam not fit with the lab findings, you would consider less obvious possibilities, including a mixed disturbance. <u>Diagnosis</u>: simple acute (uncompensated) respiratory acidosis.

Patient 9. A patient known to have stable chronic bronchitis with hypercapnia:

$$pH = 7.38 \qquad [HCO_3^-] = 31 \qquad PCO_2 = 60$$

Solution. Steps 1 & 2 indicate respiratory acidosis. PCO_2 is elevated by 20 from an assumed baseline of 40. Unless complicated by an acute exacerbation, hypercapnia associated with COPD is chronic. Use the chronic rule of thumb for Step 3: $[HCO_3^-]$ increases by 3.5–5.0 mmol/l for each 10 mm Hg rise in PCO_2. So $[HCO_3^-]$ is predicted to rise 7–10 mmol/l (2 x 3.5 = 7, 2 x 5.0 = 10). Working backwards from the observed $[HCO_3^-]$ of 31, you get an assumed pre-disease baseline [HCO_3^-] of $21-24$ ($31-10=21$, $31-7=24$). Again, the picture fits together: a chronic stable PCO_2 of 60 that is appropriately compensated by an [HCO_3^-] of 31, which rose from a pre-disease normal level of between 21 and 24. Notice that pH is in the normal range. As mentioned in Chapter 5 (p. 56), compensation for respiratory disturbances (both alkalosis and acidosis) can bring pH into the normal range, though it will not normally return pH all the way to its original baseline set point. Therefore, if the observed pH had been 7.4 (the assumed baseline) instead of 7.38, you would have seriously considered the possibility of a mixed disturbance. Diagnosis: simple chronic (compensated) respiratory acidosis.

Patient 10. A patient with several days of severe diarrhea:

$$pH = 7.15 \qquad [HCO_3^-] = 12 \qquad PCO_2 = 36$$

Solution. Steps 1 & 2 tell you that metabolic acidosis is present—consistent with the history (since diarrhea can cause metabolic acidosis). Using the Winters' formula for Step 3, you see that PCO_2 is much higher than predicted.* It appears that some defect in the respiratory system is preventing adequate compensation. In other words, a respiratory acidosis is likely superimposed on the metabolic acidosis (i.e., a mixed metabolic acidosis and respiratory acidosis is present). If the patient's history or physical exam also suggests a respiratory impairment, your diagnosis is strengthened. Still, you recognize it is possible that not enough time has elapsed for compensation to fully develop, accounting for the high PCO_2 without there being a respiratory acidosis. This possibility seems unlikely, since the diarrhea has persisted for several days and you know that respiratory compensation reaches its final level in 12–24 hours. (As mentioned on page 130, compensation for metabolic disturbances usually develops in tandem with the underlying disturbance). Nonetheless, it is possible there was a marked decline in [HCO_3^-] during the last day, so perhaps compensation has not yet caught up with that most recent incremental decrease in [HCO_3^-]. Bottom line: a metabolic acidosis with a superimposed respiratory acidosis is very likely, but a simple, not-yet-fully compensated metabolic acidosis remains a possibility. Diagnosis (tentative): mixed metabolic acidosis and respiratory acidosis.

Patient 11. An acutely ill patient with a new-onset visual impairment and a history of alcoholism and other substance abuse. The patient is breathing deeply and rapidly.

$$pH = 7.38 \qquad [HCO_3^-] = 12 \qquad PCO_2 = 21$$

Solution. Steps 1 & 2 indicate metabolic acidosis. The history of alcoholism/substance abuse and the finding of impaired vision makes you suspect methanol ingestion, since methanol can damage the optic nerve. The breathing pattern and low PCO_2 both suggest hyperventilation, which in this patient is likely respiratory compensation for the metabolic acidosis. Using the Winters' formula for Step 3, you

---

* **Hint.** Here's the math for the Winters' formula: $1.5 \times 12 = 18$. $18 + 8 = 26$. $26 \pm 2 = 24-28$ mm Hg.

see that PCO_2 is lower than expected, indicating a greater level of hyperventilation than you'd expect based on compensation alone.* This suggests a superimposed respiratory alkalosis. Two likely possible causes for the respiratory alkalosis in this patient are liver disease from chronic alcoholism and sepsis due to infection. Regardless of the particular cause, the blood gas suggests that a pathological reduction of PCO_2 (respiratory alkalosis) is superimposed on the compensatory change in PCO_2. <u>Diagnosis:</u> mixed metabolic acidosis and respiratory alkalosis. <u>Note:</u> Even before checking the rule of thumb in Step 3, you could have noticed that pH was in the normal range. Yet you know that compensation for a simple metabolic disturbance does not return pH to the normal range. Thus, even before Step 3, you could know that an additional disturbance lowered PCO_2 below its expected value and thus raised pH into the normal range. You didn't even need to do Step 3 to diagnose the mixed disturbance.

> **Patient 12.** A child in status asthmaticus (a severe, acute asthmatic episode) comes to the emergency room. The mother says the episode started several hours ago
>
> pH = 7.24 $[HCO_3^-]$ = 26 PCO_2 = 65

Solution. Steps 1 & 2 point to respiratory acidosis. The history suggests an acute episode, so for Step 3 you use the acute rule of thumb. Compensation is as predicted.** <u>Diagnosis:</u> acute (uncompensated) respiratory acidosis.

> **Patient 13.** This case follows directly from the previous one (Patient 12). Later the same day, a woman with a history of chronic bronchitis comes to the emergency room. The blood gas is identical to that of the asthmatic child: pH = 7.24, $[HCO_3^-]$ = 26, PCO_2 = 65. The woman has no fever or cyanosis, and she tells you that her sputum production is no heavier than usual. Pause here and try to formulate a possible explanation for the blood gas, then keep reading. As you are speaking with the woman, she urgently has to use the toilet. When she returns, she tells you that she has had diarrhea for several days. Her skin turgor is poor, suggesting volume depletion. Explain the blood gas in light of the history and physical exam findings.

Solution. Steps 1 & 2 indicate respiratory acidosis. Step 3: As with the asthmatic child, the blood gas is consistent with an acute disturbance, with $[HCO_3^-]$ just a couple of mmol/l above the midpoint of the normal range. But you know that COPD, especially chronic bronchitis, often causes *chronic* hypercapnia. You check the woman's chart and find that her baseline PCO_2 is, in fact, chronically elevated, with

---

* **Hint.** 1.5 x 12 = 18. 18 + 8 = 26. 26 ± 2 = 24–28 mm Hg.

** **Hint.** According to the rule, a 25 mm Hg increase in PCO_2 should raise $[HCO_3^-]$ by about 2.5 mmol/l, which is consistent with the observed value of 26, assuming an initial $[HCO_3^-]$ of 23–24 mmol/l. Since this assumed initial $[HCO_3^-]$ is well within the normal range, the picture fits together.

renal compensation in place (i.e., her baseline $[HCO_3^-]$ is appropriately elevated). Now the story becomes clear. The woman had chronic (compensated) hypercapnia and then developed metabolic acidosis from diarrhea, which reduced $[HCO_3^-]$ into the normal range—a mixed disturbance. <u>Diagnosis</u>: chronic respiratory acidosis with a superimposed metabolic acidosis. This case emphasizes two important points. First, the blood gas always must be interpreted in light of available history and physical exam information. Second, mixed disturbances sometimes produce blood gas profiles that, at first glance, look like simple disturbances.*

> **Patient 14.** A young man, still slightly intoxicated following a two-day binge of intense drinking and heavy vomiting:
>
> pH = 7.39 $[HCO_3^-]$ = 22 PCO_2 = 38

Solution. The blood gas is normal. In fact, this is the same, completely normal blood gas given for Patient 5 earlier in this chapter. But the history makes you suspicious that something more complex is going on. <u>Likely diagnosis</u>: a mixed disturbance consisting of alcoholic ketoacidosis (metabolic acidosis) and metabolic alkalosis from vomiting (p. 121). The alcoholic ketoacidosis likely reduced $[HCO_3^-]$, and the metabolic alkalosis likely raised it back to a normal level. Put differently, the opposing influences on $[HCO_3^-]$ are approximately equal. This example again emphasizes the importance of interpreting laboratory data in light of the history and physical examination. Additional lab tests (such as the anion gap, discussed in the next chapter) might confirm your suspicion, but the history itself is highly suggestive.

Rules of Thumb: User Beware

Now that you have a practical foundation in blood gas interpretation, I need to give you an important qualification and caveat. Rules of thumb are based on imperfect studies that are of only approximate relevance to any particular patient. Even the "plus/minus" (±) allowances and ranges built into the rules do not fully adjust for the imprecision. Furthermore, in the most severe acid base disturbances—in which the blood gas values lie at the very high or low extremes—the rules of thumb become less accurate. *For all these reasons, it is best to think of the formulas not as actual "rules" but, instead, as moderately flexible "guides."* Rather than focusing on absolute numerical cutoffs between simple and mixed disturbances, focus on levels of suspicion: the further the compensatory value is from the middle region of the predicted range, the more you should consider the possibility of a mixed disturbance.

---

* **Clinical note.** To get a sense of how severe the metabolic acidosis might be in this patient, you can subtract her current $[HCO_3^-]$ from the baseline compensated level recorded in her chart. For example, if the chart showed a baseline of 35 mmol/l, you could estimate that her bicarbonate level fell 9 mmol/l (35 − 26 = 9) due to the metabolic acidosis. In a patient without chronic respiratory acidosis, $[HCO_3^-]$ would have been around 15 mmol/l (24 − 9 = 15).

Summary

ABG normal values (and ranges) are pH = 7.4 (7.35–7.45), PCO_2 = 40 mm Hg (35–45), and $[HCO_3^-]$ = 24 mmol/l (21–27). The blood gas reflects two distinct processes: the disturbance and the compensation. Compensation may be present, absent, or partial, depending on how much time has passed since the disturbance developed. Compensation develops fully in a predictable period: 12–24 hours for metabolic disturbances, 3–5 days for respiratory disturbances. Metabolic disturbances usually develop gradually, thus giving the compensation, which arises relatively rapidly, time to develop in tandem; as a result, these patients are usually compensated by the time they present. In contrast, respiratory disturbances, because they compensate more slowly, often have distinct acute (uncompensated) or chronic (compensated) blood gas profiles. You can approach blood gas diagnosis in three steps. Step 1: Look at pH. Acidemia implies acidosis. Alkalemia implies alkalosis. Step 2: Determine whether the "-osis" is metabolic or respiratory by evaluating $[HCO_3^-]$ and PCO_2. The goal is to see which of these two variables can account for the *direction* of the pH change. In a simple, compensated disturbance, the variable that cannot account for the direction of the pH change will follow the same-direction rule. That is, the compensatory variable will be deviated in the same direction as the primary variable (e.g., a *high* $[HCO_3^-]$ will be accompanied by a *high* PCO_2). If both $[HCO_3^-]$ and PCO_2 can independently account for the direction of the pH change, a mixed disturbance is present. Step 3: Use the appropriate rule of thumb to find the predicted numerical value for the compensatory variable. If the observed compensation is not as predicted, a mixed disturbance is likely.

Chapter 12

Diagnosis with Venous Bicarbonate, Anion Gap, and Potassium

The arterial blood gas (ABG), which we studied in Chapter 11, gets a lot of attention. It is sometimes considered the gold standard of acid-base diagnosis. But because ABGs are relatively invasive—typically, a needle is inserted into the radial artery—you will not get a blood gas for all patients or in all situations. For this reason, simple venous blood tests (so-called "blood chemistries"), which are commonly ordered on all acutely ill patients, will often be your primary means of detecting and diagnosing acid-base disorders. Frequently, you will order these venous tests as part of a "panel," such as the SMA-7, that comprises several tests.* Even when you do get an ABG, tracking the venous chemistries over time may eliminate the need for repeating the blood gas.

Some tests in the venous panel are relevant for identifying *underlying conditions* that can cause acid-base disturbances. Examples are creatinine (e.g., renal failure) and glucose (e.g., DKA). However, it is the four electrolytes (ions) on the panel—Na^+, K^+, Cl^-, HCO_3^-—that have the broadest relevance for acid-base diagnosis. The bicarbonate level ($[HCO_3^-]$) and the anion gap (which is calculated from the electrolytes) are especially important, and they are the focus of this chapter. The plasma potassium level ($[K^+]$) sometimes gives additional clues for acid-base diagnosis, so I say a few words about $[K^+]$ as well. Your overall goal for this chapter is to learn how to get as much acid-base information as possible from the venous electrolytes, even when you don't have a blood gas or other test results. For this reason, I say relatively little here about ABGs and other tests.

Venous [HCO₃-]—Usually Measured as "Total CO₂"

In most hospitals, when you order a venous chemistry panel, a funny thing happens: the lab report does *not* list "bicarbonate concentration" or "$[HCO_3^-]$" as one of the results. Instead, it says "Total CO_2." Some labs shorten this to "TCO_2" or "CO_2" (with no "P" in front) or the words "carbon dioxide." This terminology is

---

* **Terminology.** The simplest venous chemistry panel—often called an SMA-7, SMAC-7, or Chem-7—consists of seven separate tests done on the same blood sample: BUN, creatinine, glucose, and the four common electrolytes (Na^+, K^+, Cl^-, HCO_3^-). The BMP (Basic Metabolic Panel) adds Ca^{2+} to these seven.

used because most labs assess venous $[HCO_3^-]$ with a technique that simultaneously measures bicarbonate and several other substances that have a CO_2 built into their chemical formulas. (To see the CO_2 in bicarbonate, mentally delete the H and one of the O's from HCO_3^-.) The measured sum of these CO_2-related substances is referred to as Total CO_2.

The non-bicarbonate substances included in Total CO_2 are present in very low concentrations. Taken together, they increase the numerical value for Total CO_2 by roughly 5 percent above the actual venous $[HCO_3^-]$. At a normal plasma $[HCO_3^-]$, this 5 percent translates into a bit less than 1.5 mmol/liter. This small difference is usually inconsequential and, as a practical matter, *you can consider Total CO_2 as being equal to actual $[HCO_3^-]$*. In fact, many clinicians use the terms "Total CO_2" and "venous $[HCO_3^-]$" interchangeably. In this chapter, both terms are used—sometimes one, and sometimes the other—so you can get used to both.*

The normal range for venous $[HCO_3^-]$, measured as Total CO_2, is about 23–29 mmol/l, with a midpoint of 26. This range and midpoint is about 2 mmol/l higher than for arterial $[HCO_3^-]$ (p. 125). Two factors account for this 2 mmol/l difference. The most important is the presence of non-bicarbonate substances in the venous Total CO_2 measurement. As mentioned, these usually account for just under 1.5 mmol/l. The second, minor factor is that normal venous blood has a slightly higher PCO_2 than arterial blood (typically 46 vs. 40 mm Hg). The higher PCO_2 shifts the equilibrium of $CO_2 + H_2O \leftrightharpoons H^+ + HCO_3^-$ in plasma slightly to the right, raising venous $[HCO_3^-]$ by about 0.5 mmol/l.

Total CO_2 a.k.a. venous $[HCO_3^-]$ = 26 (23–29) mmol/l

vs.

Arterial $[HCO_3^-]$ = 24 (21–27) mmol/l

Metabolic acid-base disturbances affect $[HCO_3^-]$ *directly* and respiratory acid-base disturbances affect $[HCO_3^-]$ *indirectly*, via renal compensation, as predicted by the same-direction rule (p. 55). As a result, most acid-base disturbances alter $[HCO_3^-]$. In fact, the only acid-base disturbances that don't markedly alter venous $[HCO_3^-]$ are (1) acute (uncompensated) respiratory disturbances ($[HCO_3^-]$ changes by just a little) and (2) certain mixed disturbances that have opposing effects on $[HCO_3^-]$, such as an equal-strength metabolic acidosis and alkalosis. Therefore, venous $[HCO_3^-]$—Total CO_2—can tell you a lot. A low Total CO_2 indicates either a metabolic acidosis or a compensated respiratory alkalosis. A high Total CO_2 indicates either a metabolic alkalosis or a compensated respiratory acidosis. To start applying these ideas, try a few clinical examples:

---

*__Going further.__ The non-bicarbonate substances in Total CO_2 include carbonic acid (H_2CO_3), the carbonate anion (CO_3^{2-}), and CO_2 itself, either as dissolved CO_2 gas in the plasma or as CO_2 bound to hemoglobin and other blood proteins (the so-called "carbamino compounds"). Of the non-bicarbonate substances measured in TCO_2, dissolved CO_2 gas is by far the largest component.

Patient 1. A child with insulin-dependent diabetes presents with dehydration, a recent history of polyuria and polydipsia, and a venous [HCO_3^-] of 14.

Solution. The bicarbonate value itself could represent either metabolic acidosis or compensated respiratory alkalosis. In light of the history and physical exam, metabolic acidosis (diabetic ketoacidosis) is almost certain.

Patient 2. A previously healthy woman presents with a G.I infection and three days of vomiting. Total CO_2 is 36.

Solution. An elevated Total CO_2 can represent either metabolic alkalosis or chronic (compensated) respiratory acidosis. The history points to metabolic alkalosis.

Patient 3. A long-time smoker with COPD and known stable hypercapnia has an [HCO_3^-] of 33 and no other unusual findings.

Solution 3. Given the history, this patient has a compensated respiratory acidosis, not metabolic alkalosis.

These three patients illustrate how a Total CO_2, in conjunction with key historical and physical exam findings, may be all you need to make a correct diagnosis. But sometimes more information is required, as these next two patients illustrate:

Patient 4. A woman with COPD presents with fever, cyanosis, and a TCO_2 of 32.

Solution. Is the elevated Total CO_2 explained by renal compensation for chronic hypercapnia? Possibly, but we don't know if this COPD patient is normally hypercapnic (not all are, even among those with chronic bronchitis). Alternatively, fever in a COPD patient raises the possibility of a respiratory infection, which might be increasing PCO_2 acutely from a non-hypercapnic baseline. Or maybe the patient normally has marked hypercapnia and a compensated [HCO_3^-] of, say, 37—which has been reduced to 32 by an acute metabolic acidosis, perhaps lactic acidosis from hypoxemia (note the cyanosis). More information—probably including a blood gas—is needed.

Patient 5. A chronically hospitalized patient with intermittent diarrhea has a venous [HCO_3^-] of 17.

Solution. Is this metabolic acidosis from diarrhea? Or is the metabolic acidosis from another cause? Or does the low [HCO_3^-] represent the compensation for chronic respiratory alkalosis from undiagnosed hypoxemia or liver disease? We can't be sure. More information is needed.*

---

* **Clinical note.** Venous TCO_2 from the chemistry panel, and arterial [HCO_3^-] from the ABG, give you essentially the same information—bicarbonate status—with slightly different normal ranges. Therefore, if you have a timely measure of one, you don't need the other. The specific clinical value of TCO_2 arises from its being less invasive to obtain, so you'll often have freer access to TCO_2 than to arterial [HCO_3^-]. However, if you have easy access to arterial blood—say, in an ICU patient who has an arterial line (catheter) in place from which you can obtain the arterial blood sample directly without further punctures—there is no need to measure TCO_2 at all. You can even measure blood chemistries, and calculate the anion gap, from the arterial sample.

Anion Gap

The Anion Gap Concept

The law of electroneutrality tells you that blood plasma, like all solutions, contains an equal number of positive and negative charges. It follows that if you graphically stack up plasma cations (positively charged ions) and anions (negatively charged ions) side by side, the resulting "ionogram" will have two columns of equal height. Scan this figure, then keep reading:

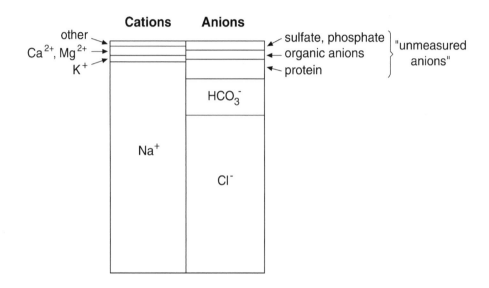

The height of the columns indicates the total ion concentrations, measured in equivalents (i.e., the concentration of *charges*). Looking at the figure, notice that the major cation is Na^+. The minor cations include K^+, Ca^{2+}, and Mg^{2+}. The major anions are Cl^- and HCO_3^-. The minor anions include sulfate, phosphate, organic acid anions such as lactate and acetoacetate, as well as the negative charges on plasma proteins (especially albumin). Of the various plasma anions, only Cl^- and HCO_3^- are *routinely* measured in the hospital laboratory. For this reason, all the other anions are sometimes lumped together and called "**unmeasured anions**." Take a moment to notice that important label on the figure.

Consider a patient who has metabolic acidosis due to the addition of strong acid. What happens to the ionogram in this situation? (Refer to the above ionogram as you continue to read, visualizing the changes with your mind's eye.) First, the strong acid releases protons. These protons are buffered by bicarbonate, via the reaction $H^+ + HCO_3^- \rightarrow CO_2 + H_2O$. This reaction causes plasma $[HCO_3^-]$ to decrease, shrinking the $[HCO_3^-]$ region of the ionogram. Second, the anions from the dissociated strong acid are added to the plasma. Depending on the type of acid, the anion will expand either the Cl^- region or the "unmeasured anion" region of the ionogram. For example, if hydrochloric acid (HCl) is added to the plasma, $[Cl^-]$ rises and the Cl^- region of the ionogram expands. If lactic acid is added to blood plasma, [lactate] rises and the unmeasured anion region of the ionogram expands. In fact, if any acid *other* than HCl is added to blood plasma, the unmeasured anion region expands.*

In summary: *when acid enters the plasma, the bicarbonate region shrinks due to buffering, and the vacated space in the anion column is filled by the expansion of either unmeasured anions or Cl⁻.* This expansion maintains the height of the anion column and, with it, the electroneutrality of the blood plasma. The following three ionograms fully illustrate these points. Study these ionograms and then keep reading.

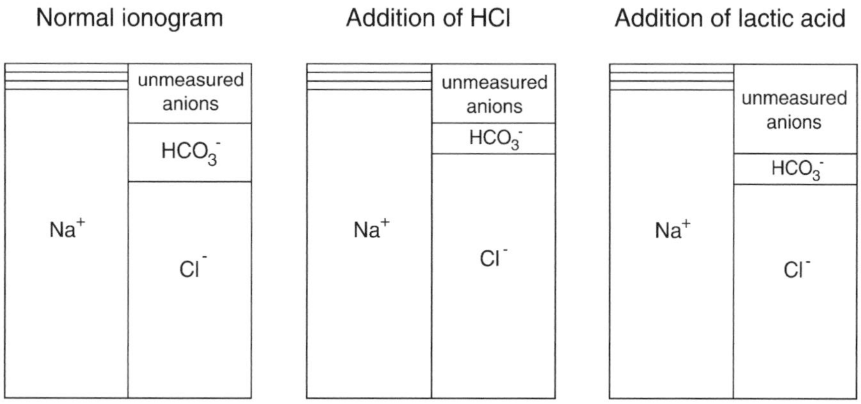

Normal ionogram	Addition of HCl	Addition of lactic acid

Notice that the ionogram on the left portrays the normal or baseline situation. The middle ionogram reflects the addition of HCl, which expands the Cl^- region. The ionogram on the right represents the addition of lactic acid, which expands the unmeasured anion region. As mentioned above, any acid other than HCl expands the unmeasured anion region. In the middle and right ionograms, notice that the bicarbonate region is smaller than normal. This is what you expect, since acid has been added in both cases. Be sure these points all make sense to you before proceeding.

You may be wondering why I keep talking about adding HCl to the blood plasma. Obviously, you won't normally encounter patients who have ingested or been infused with hydrochloric acid. The HCl ionogram is important because it is the same ionogram as occurs with metabolic acidosis associated with diarrhea and several other important causes of metabolic acidosis. In these conditions, HCl is not actually added to the body, but plasma $[HCO_3^-]$ decreases and additional Cl^- is retained by the kidney, so $[Cl^-]$ rises. The net effect is *as if* HCl had been added, so the ionogram looks the same.

Now consider a patient with metabolic acidosis of unknown cause. If you could see the patient's ionogram, you would gain valuable diagnostic information. If the ionogram looked like the one on the right in the above figure, you would suspect the acidosis was of a type that leaves an anion other than chloride (e.g., lactic acidosis, ketoacidosis). If the ionogram looked like the one in the middle, you would suspect a different set of causes, including diarrhea.

---

*__Hint.__ All anions in the plasma other than HCO_3^- are either Cl^- or "unmeasured." In addition, the anions of all strong acids are either Cl^- or unmeasured. Therefore, any strong acid added to the body will raise either $[Cl^-]$ or [unmeasured anions].

In reality, clinicians cannot routinely get enough information to construct a complete ionogram. However, it's possible to construct a *simplified* ionogram by assuming that (1) Na⁺ is the only cation in plasma and (2) the anion column is only as tall as the Na⁺ column. (These assumptions aren't too bad, since Na⁺ is by far the most prevalent cation in the plasma.) The assumptions have the effect of "decapitating" the ionogram at the top of the Na⁺ column, like this:

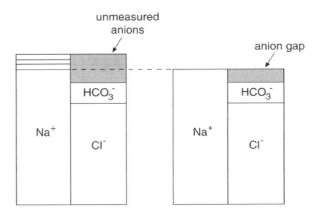

What interests us most in the simplified ionogram is the region labeled "**anion gap**." Although the anion gap region of the decapitated (simplified) ionogram is smaller than the unmeasured anion region of the full ionogram, *the sizes of the two regions change in parallel.* Thus, when the concentration of unmeasured anions is normal, the anion gap is of normal size. When the concentration of unmeasured anions increases, the anion gap gets bigger. The clinical importance of this will become clear soon. Study the following "table" for a moment, then continue to read:

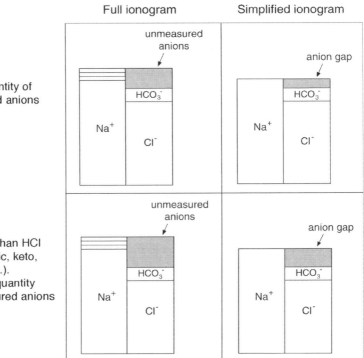

This graphic "table" shows two patients who have a low plasma $[HCO_3^-]$ due to the addition of acid. In the top row, the acid was HCl, which increased $[Cl^-]$ and left [unmeasured anions] unchanged. In the bottom row, the acid was one such as lactic acid or a keto acid, which increased [unmeasured anions] but left $[Cl^-]$ unchanged. The left column shows the complete ionograms and hence the total concentrations of unmeasured anions. The right column shows the decapitated ionograms and hence the anion gaps. Notice that when the unmeasured anion region expands (bottom left), the anion gap region expands with it (bottom right). Make sure all aspects of this table make sense to you.

We now arrive at a key point. Look at either of the simplified ionograms (right column) in the above figure. Notice that the size of the anion gap is equal to the height of the Na^+ column minus the combined heights of the HCO_3^- and Cl^- regions. We can thus describe the size of the anion gap region by using a simple formula:

$$\text{Anion gap} = [Na^+] - ([Cl^-] + [HCO_3^-])$$

This formula is invaluable. It lets you use readily available lab data ($[Na^+]$, $[Cl^-]$, and $[HCO_3^-]$) to calculate the size of the anion gap. And knowing the size of the gap lets you assess whether the quantity of unmeasured anions is normal or elevated. You do not have to draw an ionogram or even a decapitated ionogram. You can figure it all out with numbers using the above formula. For practice, find the anion gap in the following four patients. Although it's usual to write "$[HCO_3^-]$" in the gap formula, normal ranges for the anion are actually determined using the venous Total CO_2 values. Therefore, you should use the Total CO_2 values when you calculate the gap.*

> **Patient 6.** $[Na^+] = 140\,\text{mmol/l}$, $[Cl^-] = 105\,\text{mmol/l}$, $[HCO_3^-] = 25$ mmol/l
>
> **Patient 7.** $[Na^+] = 140$, $[Cl^-] = 100$, $[HCO_3^-] = 15$
>
> **Patient 8.** $[Na^+] = 138$, $[Cl^-] = 98$, and $[HCO_3^-] = 24$
>
> **Patient 9.** $[Na^+] = 145$, $[Cl^-] = 105$, and $[HCO_3^-] = 11$
>
> *Answers:* 10, 25, 16, 29

The **normal range** for the anion gap varies *markedly* among laboratories, depending on the type of blood analysis machine and how it is calibrated. In many hospitals, the normal range is 8 to 16 (i.e., 12 ± 4) and that's the normal range we'll use in this book. However, in your clinical work it is *essential* that you know the normal range in your particular hospital or lab. Depending on the lab, the normal range can be as much as 5 units (milliequivalents per liter) lower than the range we will be working with.

Clinical note. Although using venous blood is preferable, the error introduced by using an arterial sample is relatively small. This makes it possible to run blood chemistries, and calculate the anion gap, using an arterial sample when the patient already has an arterial line in place, as discussed in the footnote on page 139.

> Normal anion gap = 8–16 (12 ± 4)
> Varies from lab to lab—learn yours!

Using the Anion Gap Clinically

Let's start with terminology. During metabolic acidosis, the decrease in $[HCO_3^-]$ is always accompanied by an increase in the concentration of either unmeasured anions or chloride. Based on this fact, two general presentations of metabolic acidosis can be distinguished. When unmeasured anion concentration rises, the anion gap enlarges and, therefore, the acidosis is called an **anion gap metabolic acidosis**. When $[Cl^-]$ increases, the anion gap does not enlarge and, therefore, the acidosis is called a **non-anion gap metabolic acidosis**.*

Different causes of metabolic acidosis are associated with one or the other of these two presentations. A gap greater than 16 (or the upper limit of your lab's normal range) suggests one of the anion gap causes. In fact, if the gap is in the high end of the normal range, you should at least consider the possibility that the patient's baseline gap was actually low-normal, and that the seemingly normal (high-normal) gap actually represents a modest increase. Three conditions account for most cases of anion gap metabolic acidosis:

- ketoacidosis
- lactic acidosis
- renal failure

The next most common cause of anion gap metabolic acidosis is toxic ingestion with methanol, ethylene glycol, or salicylates.** Conversely, a normal gap suggests one of the non-gap causes. As with gap acidosis, three conditions account for most cases of non-gap metabolic acidosis:

- diarrhea
- renal failure
- renal tubular acidosis (RTA)

Renal failure is listed in both the gap and non-gap categories because it can present with either a normal or elevated gap. The gap presentation is more common when renal failure is severe (reflected in a markedly elevated creatinine level). RTA is less common than the other two causes; it is usually first suspected when a non-gap metabolic acidosis cannot be attributed to either diarrhea or renal failure.

---

* **Terminology.** Anion gap metabolic acidosis is also known as "normochloremic metabolic acidosis" because the blood chloride level is normal. Similarly, non-anion gap metabolic acidosis is also known as "hyperchloremic metabolic acidosis" because the chloride level is increased. Note that when you say "non-gap metabolic acidosis," you're really using a shorthand for "*non-elevated* gap acidosis," in that the gap is normal (e.g., 8–16), not zero.

** **Mnemonic.** MEG'S LARD gives the common causes of gap acidosis. MEG'S lists the most common toxic ingestions: Methanol, Ethylene Glycol, Salicylate. LARD lists the non-intoxicant causes: Lactic acidosis, Alcoholic ketoacidosis, Renal failure, Diabetic ketoacidosis.

Before going further, take a moment to study the following table, which summarizes basic information about the most common gap and non-gap causes of metabolic acidosis. Give a bit of special attention to the third column, which provides some clinically useful information not discussed elsewhere in the text: the largest gap size commonly encountered for each of the main causes of gap acidosis.

Gap and Non-Gap Causes of Metabolic Acidosis		
Cause	Predominant Anions	Maximum Gap Size, Approximate*
Ketoacidosis— Both diabetic (DKA) and alcoholic (AKA)	Keto-acid anions (Acetoacetate, beta-hydroxybutyrate)	35–40
Lactic acidosis	Lactate	>35
Renal failure	Sulfate, phosphate, urate, hippurate. In non-gap presentation: chloride	25. Can also present with a normal anion gap
Toxic Ingestion— Especially salicylate, ethylene glycol, and methanol	Formate, glycolate, glycoaldehyde, glyoxylate, oxalate, keto-acid anions	Salicylate 20–30 Ethylene glycol > 35 Methanol > 35
Diarrhea	Chloride	Non-gap
Renal Tubular Acidosis	Chloride	Non-gap

*Note the word "maximum." The numbers in this column are the highest you're likely to encounter for each cause of gap acidosis. All causes of gap acidosis can present with gap values that are only slightly elevated. A gap of up to 25 can indicate any cause of gap acidosis.

Try this problem:

Patient 10. $[Na^+] = 146$, $[Cl^-] = 104$, $[HCO_3^-] = 9$. What is the anion gap? For practice, list by memory all the common causes of gap metabolic acidosis. Based simply on the numerical value of the gap in this patient, which potential causes of gap acidosis are *not* likely? For additional practice, list the most common causes of non-gap metabolic acidosis.

Solution. The anion gap is 33. Common gap causes: ketoacidosis (AKA and DKA), lactic acidosis, renal failure (especially when severe), methanol, ethylene glycol, salicylates. Renal failure and salicylates are unlikely. Most common non-gap causes: diarrhea, renal failure, renal tubular acidosis.

Anion Gap in Mixed Disturbances

The anion gap helps you determine the cause of metabolic acidosis. For this reason, a common sequence is this: You look at the venous electrolytes, notice a low Total CO_2, and then check the anion gap. This sequence is appropriate. However, even if Total CO_2 is normal or elevated, *you still must check the gap*. The reason: If an anion gap metabolic acidosis is mixed with a bicarbonate-raising process (either a metabolic alkalosis or a compensated respiratory acidosis—these are the only two possibilities), then Total CO_2 can be normal or elevated but the gap will remain high. If the bicarbonate-raising process is equal in magnitude to the metabolic acidosis, $[HCO_3^-]$ will be normal. If the bicarbonate-raising process is of greater magnitude than the metabolic acidosis, $[HCO_3^-]$ will be elevated. In either case, the gap will still be high—a telltale indication of an otherwise invisible anion gap metabolic acidosis. Try these two problems:

Patient 11. $[Na^+] = 142$, $[Cl^-] = 96$, $[HCO_3^-] = 24$

Solution. The gap is 22 and Total CO_2 is normal (instead of decreased). This combination suggests a mixed disturbance: an anion gap metabolic acidosis and an equal-strength bicarbonate-raising process (metabolic alkalosis or compensated respiratory acidosis).

Patient 12. $[Na^+] = 146$, $[Cl^-] = 89$, $[HCO_3^-] = 31$

Solution. The gap is elevated and TCO_2 is elevated (instead of decreased). This combination suggests a mixed disturbance: a gap metabolic acidosis and a more-than-offsetting bicarbonate-raising process (metabolic alkalosis or compensated respiratory acidosis).

When you encounter lab values like these last two sets, you'll try to decide if the bicarbonate-raising processes is metabolic alkalosis or compensated respiratory acidosis. The history and physical exam will often clarify the situation. For instance, if the patient has severe renal failure (gap metabolic acidosis), no history of chronic lung disease, and has been vomiting heavily, you'll know that the bicarbonate-raising process is metabolic alkalosis.

The Anion Gap in Blood Gas Interpretation

Just as you'll check the anion gap whenever you get a venous chemistry panel, you should check the anion gap whenever you get a blood gas. If you want, you can think of checking the anion gap as an additional step (Step 4) in blood gas interpretation—added to Steps 1–3 presented in the last chapter. Try the next two problems. They will help you see how to interpret the blood gas and anion gap together:

Patient 13. pH = 7.31, $[HCO_3^-] = 13$, $PCO_2 = 27$

$[Na^+] = 141$, $[Cl^-] = 99$, Total $CO_2 = 14$

Solution. Looking at the blood gas, Steps 1–3 tell you this is a well-compensated metabolic acidosis. The anion gap is 28, indicating an anion gap metabolic acidosis.

A gap of 28 is consistent with any of the causes of gap acidosis except for renal failure, which usually has a somewhat lower gap (even when the gap is elevated at all). The history, physical exam, and other lab tests would help you decide among the possibilities.

Patient 14. pH = 7.41, [HCO$_3^-$] = 25, PCO$_2$ = 41

[Na$^+$] = 145, [Cl$^-$] = 95, Total CO$_2$ = 26

Solution. The blood gas looks completely normal. However, the anion gap is clearly elevated (24), suggesting metabolic acidosis. A bicarbonate-raising process—either metabolic alkalosis or compensated respiratory acidosis—can explain the normal [HCO$_3^-$]. Since arterial PCO$_2$ is normal, chronic respiratory acidosis is effectively ruled out, leaving metabolic alkalosis as the explanation. Had this metabolic alkalosis been dominant, [HCO$_3^-$] would have been elevated. If you hadn't checked the anion gap, you might have thought the patient had no acid-base disturbance; in fact, a mixed disturbance is present.

Potassium Level

In addition to the direct importance of plasma [K$^+$] for the patient's health (e.g., for muscle strength and cardiac rhythm), paying attention to [K$^+$] can sometimes help you make an acid-base diagnosis. In Chapters 6–9, I described how disease states that cause acid-base disorders can alter plasma [K$^+$]. The following table summarizes that information in a form useful for acid-base diagnosis. Being familiar with typical [K$^+$] values for the different causes of acid-base disturbances can increase or decrease your confidence in a suspected diagnosis. Study the table before proceeding to the practice problems.

Disturbance	Typical [K$^+$] (Normal Range = 3.5–5.0 mmol/l)
Metabolic alkalosis (all causes)	Low
Metabolic acidosis	Depends on cause, as follows—
Diarrhea	Low
Renal Failure	Usually elevated somewhat from baseline—often high normal
Renal Tubular Acidosis	Types 1 and 2: low or normal Type 4: high
Diabetic ketoacidosis, Lactic acidosis	Usually normal or high, rarely low
Alcoholic ketoacidosis, methanol, ethylene glycol, salicylates	No typical value
Respiratory disturbances	Acute: acidosis—often slightly high; alkalosis—often slightly low Chronic: normal

Practice Problems

These problems let you consider the $[HCO_3^-]$, anion gap, and $[K^+]$ together, as you would in the clinical setting. Interpret each set of labs as fully as you can before reading the solution. Assume the following normal ranges: $[HCO_3^-]$ (measured as Total CO_2) = 23–29 mmol/l, anion gap = 8–16, $[K^+]$ = 3.5–5.0 mmol/l.

Patient 15.

$[Na^+]$	=	143
$[K^+]$	=	3.3
$[Cl^-]$	=	95
$[HCO_3^-]$	=	35

Solution. The high $[HCO_3^-]$ suggests either metabolic alkalosis or compensated respiratory acidosis. The low $[K^+]$ makes metabolic alkalosis more likely, since metabolic alkalosis typically presents with hypokalemia. The normal anion gap (13) is consistent with metabolic alkalosis. A history of vomiting, nasogastric drainage, or diuretic use (the most common causes of metabolic alkalosis), would strengthen your diagnosis. If the patient is receiving mechanical ventilation, you would consider post-hypercapnic metabolic alkalosis (p. 97–98).

Patient 16.

$[Na^+]$	=	140
$[K^+]$	=	3.1
$[Cl^-]$	=	115
$[HCO_3^-]$	=	16

Solution. The low $[HCO_3^-]$ suggests either metabolic acidosis or chronic (= compensated) respiratory alkalosis. Although respiratory alkalosis can lower $[K^+]$, it does so only slightly, and even then only in *acute* (= uncompensated) respiratory alkalosis. Therefore, metabolic acidosis is more likely. (This said, you must still keep in mind that a chronic respiratory alkalosis may present with hypokalemia from a separate cause, so you should continue to hold the possibility of respiratory alkalosis in mind.) The normal anion gap (9) points away from the anion gap causes of metabolic acidosis. Of the non-gap causes, renal failure does not commonly present with hypokalemia. In contrast, diarrhea and some types of Renal Tubular Acidosis (RTA), specifically Types 1 and 2, can present with marked hypokalemia, though these RTAs are not common. If the patient gave a history of recent diarrhea, you could be reasonably confident that the diarrhea caused the acidosis. If there was no history of diarrhea, you would consider the possibility of an RTA.*

*****Clinical note.** I'm giving limited labs to work with so you can focus fully on, and learn to gain maximum information from, the four electrolytes. In a clinical situation, you'd also have a plasma creatinine level, which would let you easily rule renal failure in or out; and you could obtain a blood gas, which would let you definitively distinguish between metabolic acidosis and chronic respiratory alkalosis. One situation where a chronic respiratory alkalosis sometimes gets confused with metabolic acidosis is when a hospitalized patient has a low TCO_2, a low or normal $[K^+]$, and a normal anion gap. These patients are sometimes diagnosed with Types 1 or 2 RTA when they actually may have compensated respiratory alkalosis. Since Types 1 and 2 RTA are rare, whereas respiratory alkalosis is common in hospitalized patients, some authorities recommend getting a blood gas before entertaining one of these RTA diagnoses, especially in a hospitalized patient.

Patient 17.

$$[Na^+] = 145$$
$$[K^+] = 3.4$$
$$[Cl^-] = 81$$
$$[HCO_3^-] = 32$$

Solution. The $[HCO_3^-]$ and $[K^+]$ suggest metabolic alkalosis. But the elevated anion gap (32) suggests an anion gap metabolic acidosis. The solution is a mixed disturbance consisting of both these primary disturbances. An example here would be an alcoholic patient who experiences several days of severe vomiting (which increases $[HCO_3^-]$ and lowers $[K^+]$) and then develops alcoholic ketoacidosis. Were it not for the acidosis, which consumed some of the excess bicarbonate, plasma $[HCO_3^-]$ would be substantially higher than 32. Conversely, were it not for the metabolic alkalosis, $[HCO_3^-]$ would be very low and the lab report would have looked like a simple anion gap metabolic acidosis. Finally, if the acidosis and alkalosis had been of equal magnitudes, plasma $[HCO_3^-]$ would have been normal, though the anion gap would still be elevated.

Summary

Venous $[HCO_3^-]$, which is usually measured by the Total CO_2 assay, is low in metabolic acidosis and in compensated respiratory alkalosis, and high in metabolic alkalosis and in compensated respiratory acidosis. The anion gap, defined as $[Na^+]$ - $([Cl^-] + [HCO_3^-])$, tracks the concentration of plasma unmeasured anions. When metabolic acidosis is accompanied by an elevated anion gap, the condition is called an "anion gap metabolic acidosis" (sometimes shortened to "gap acidosis"). When metabolic acidosis is accompanied by a normal anion gap, it is called a "non-gap metabolic acidosis." The most common causes of gap acidosis are: ketoacidosis (both diabetic and alcoholic), lactic acidosis, renal failure, and toxic ingestions of methanol, ethylene glycol, or salicylates. The most common causes of non-gap acidosis are diarrhea, renal failure, and renal tubular acidosis. As comparison of the last two sentences indicates, the gap in renal failure may be either high or normal, with an elevated gap being most common when renal failure is severe, as defined by a very low glomerular filtration rate and markedly elevated plasma [creatinine]. In simple gap metabolic acidosis, the gap is high and Total CO_2 is low. If the gap is high and Total CO_2 is normal or high, a bicarbonate-raising process (either metabolic alkalosis or compensated respiratory acidosis—these are the only two possibilities) is also present (i.e., a mixed disturbance). You should calculate the anion gap even if Total CO_2 is normal or elevated. The gap should also be examined when interpreting the blood gas, even if $[HCO_3^-]$ is normal or elevated. Typical values for plasma $[K^+]$ are: low in metabolic alkalosis (regardless of cause), low in metabolic acidosis from diarrhea, high-normal or slightly elevated in renal failure, low in Types 1 and 2 RTA (though it can be normal), and high in Type 4 RTA.

Normal Values & Formulas

Venous Total CO_2 = 23–29 mmol/l

Anion gap = $[Na^+] - ([Cl^-] + [HCO_3^-])$

Normal anion gap = 8 to 16 (12 ± 4) (Varies markedly among labs)

Plasma $[K^+]$ = 3.5–5.0 mmol/l

Chapter 13

All Together Now: Integrative Problems

This chapter presents twelve diagnostic problems with detailed solutions. It forms the culmination of the book, letting you test your knowledge and see how much you've learned. The problems are integrative, incorporating various combinations of data from venous chemistries, arterial blood gases, the specific tests discussed in Chapters 6 and 7, and selected history and physical exam findings. Try to work each problem fully before checking the solution. You may find it helpful to work the problems in writing, sketching out your thought process and the various diagnostic steps and possibilities. If you need to remind yourself of any relevant factual information, feel free to look back to earlier chapters, as you would in an open-book test. Don't worry about getting the "wrong" answer: you'll still learn a great deal from the effort, and learning remains the goal even in this final chapter. Good luck and enjoy!

> **Patient 1.** A 19-year old male college student presents with fatigue and decreased muscle strength. The patient says he has not been vomiting or taking diuretics. What are the most likely possibilities?
>
> Venous chemistries: $[Na^+]$ = 145, $[Cl^-]$ = 103, $[K^+]$ = 3.0, $[HCO_3^-]$ = 34, Creatinine = 1.1, BUN = 22, glucose = 90
> Urine $[Cl^-]$ = 70 mmol/l
> No blood gas was done.

Interpretation. In the absence of obvious chronic (= compensated; p. 56) respiratory disease, the elevated plasma bicarbonate level likely represents metabolic alkalosis. The hypokalemia is consistent with this possibility, since metabolic alkalosis, regardless of the cause, usually presents with hypokalemia (p. 100, 147). The hypokalemia also likely explains the fatigue and reduced muscle strength. The high urine $[Cl^-]$ raises the possibility of volume-resistant metabolic alkalosis, since the volume-responsive causes of metabolic alkalosis, which are more common, present with a low urine $[Cl^-]$ (p. 100, 102). Primary hyperaldosteronism from either an adrenal adenoma or adrenal hyperplasia are the two most common possibilities for volume-resistant metabolic alkalosis (p. 99) and would be a logical starting point for additional workup. An elevated blood pressure would have pointed you in this direction, since primary hyperaldosteronism usually causes hypertension (p. 99). Another possibility is surreptitious diuretic use for weight loss. Since diuretics prevent urinary $[Cl^-]$ from being low even during marked volume depletion, this possibility could explain the high urine $[Cl^-]$ (p. 101). To investigate this possibility, you could repeat the labs, this time including a urine diuretic screen. If the patient had been taking diuretics but has now stopped, the screen would be negative and urine $[Cl^-]$ would be < 15 mmol/l, assuming enough time had passed for the diuretic to clear from the urine.

Patient 2. These labs are for a man in his 50s. Propose a likely diagnosis without knowing any historical or physical exam data.

ABG: pH = 7.31, $[HCO_3^-]$ = 16, PCO_2 = 33
Venous: $[Na^+]$ = 134, $[Cl^-]$ = 104, $[K^+]$ = 5.5, Total CO_2 = 17, Creatinine = 2.1, BUN = 16, glucose = 175

Interpretation. The three-step method of blood-gas interpretation (p. 126) shows a simple, appropriately compensated metabolic acidosis. The anion gap is normal, making diarrhea, non-gap renal failure, and RTA the most likely possibilities (p. 144). Diarrhea usually presents with hypokalemia (p. 69, 147), and the creatinine is too low for frank renal failure (pp. 77, 80), so you should suspect an RTA. Of the three main types of RTAs, Type 4 (a.k.a., Hyperkalemic RTA) presents with hyperkalemia and a modestly elevated creatinine (often 1.5–2 mg/dl) (p. 79). The elevated glucose raises the possibility of poorly controlled diabetes. In fact, the most common cause of Type 4 RTA is hyporeninemic hypoaldosteronism (a low plasma [aldosterone] secondary to impaired renin secretion by the kidney) resulting from diabetic nephropathy (p. 79). This possibility should be explored further.

Patient 3. A pregnant woman, mid-third trimester, comes in for a regular prenatal check up. She reports several months of mild dyspnea when doing light physical activity. She says the dyspnea is now sometimes present at rest. What's the likely explanation and what else do you need to worry about?

Venous labs: $[Na^+]$ = 140, $[Cl^-]$ = 107, $[K^+]$ = 4.6, Total CO_2 = 19
Lungs are clear on physical exam. Oxygen saturation by pulse oximetry is 98 percent. She has no history of asthma.

Interpretation. The most likely explanation for both the low Total CO_2 and the mild dyspnea is the mild, chronic (= compensated) respiratory alkalosis that typically accompanies normal pregnancy (p. 119). Nonetheless, you need to consider the possibility of pulmonary disease, especially pulmonary embolism and asthma. In contrast to the dyspnea of pregnancy, which has a gradual onset, dyspnea from pulmonary embolism usually has an acute onset and may be associated with pleuritic chest pain and hemoptysis, findings not present in normal pregnancy. Asthma would be suggested by a prior history of asthma, wheezing on chest exam, and obstruction during pulmonary function tests. A cough, which is not usually present in pregnancy, might suggest a primary lung or cardiac cause for the dyspnea.

Patient 4. An acutely ill patient is brought to the emergency department. Venous and arterial blood is immediately drawn.

Venous: $[Na^+]$ = 136, $[Cl^-]$ = 103, $[K^+]$ = 5.5, Total CO_2 = 15

ABG: pH = 7.32, [HCO$_3^-$] = 19, PCO$_2$ = 34
What acid-base disorder is present? Do you notice any inconsistencies in these lab results?

Interpretation. The lab tests point to metabolic acidosis, but you should recognize that inconsistencies (and hence possible lab errors) are present. First, Total CO$_2$ does not closely match arterial [HCO$_3^-$]. The values usually match within about 2 mmol/l (p. 138)—but here they are 4 mmol/l apart. Second—and exacerbating the first inconsistency—the patient's arterial [HCO$_3^-$] is higher than venous Total CO$_2$, the reverse of what you should expect. TCO$_2$ should always be (slightly) higher than arterial [HCO$_3^-$] since (a) the TCO$_2$ assay measures bicarbonate plus several other minor substances and (b) venous PCO$_2$ is normally slightly higher than arterial (typically about 6 mm Hg higher; p. 32, 138). Thus, in venous blood the CO$_2$ + H$_2$O $\rightleftharpoons$ H$^+$ + HCO$_3^-$ equilibrium is displaced slightly to the right, raising [HCO$_3^-$] slightly (p. 138). These inconsistencies, and the lab errors they may reflect, introduce uncertainty into your acid-base diagnosis; you therefore may want to repeat one or both of the labs.*

Patient 5. A 45-year old man is brought semi-conscious to the emergency room. A family member tells you he was despondent last night and may have ingested a toxin or deliberately overdosed with some medication. What do the history and lab results point to?

Venous: [Na$^+$] = 140, [Cl$^-$] = 100, [K$^+$] = 4.0, Total CO$_2$ = 14
ABG: pH = 7.48, [HCO$_3^-$] = 13, PCO$_2$ = 18

Interpretation. Looking at the ABG, Steps 1 and 2 indicate a respiratory alkalosis. For Step 3, you need to decide which rule of thumb to apply. The low [HCO$_3^-$] could make you think this is a compensated respiratory alkalosis. In fact, the numerical value of [HCO$_3^-$] is not far from what you'd expect based on the chronic respiratory alkalosis rule of thumb (a 4 mmol/l decrement in [HCO$_3^-$] for each 10 mm Hg decrement in PCO$_2$; pp. 64, 130.) However, the current illness developed just last night, ruling out a chronic respiratory disorder. Therefore, the respiratory alkalosis must be acute (= uncompensated; p. 56) or very nearly so. The [HCO$_3^-$] must therefore be low because of a superimposed metabolic acidosis. The anion gap is elevated. Salicylates can cause a mixed disturbance: an anion gap metabolic acidosis and respiratory alkalosis (p. 75). A toxic level on the plasma salicylate assay would confirm the diagnosis, though a low level of salicylate might merely indicate that the patient recently used aspirin, or an aspirin-containing product, for pain relief.

---

*Going further.** This footnote gives an optional teaching point for more advanced students. An additional problem with the labs reveals itself if you check the blood gas for *internal consistency.* Here's how to check. Starting with the second H-H equation on p. 25, replace the [CO$_2$] term with (PCO$_2$ x 0.03), like this: pH = 6.1 + log ([HCO$_3^-$]/(PCO$_2$ x 0.03)). Because it incorporates the CO$_2$ solubility constant (p. 17), this form of the H-H lets you plug PCO$_2$ values directly into the equation. Now, plug the PCO$_2$ and [HCO$_3^-$] values from the blood gas into this H-H and, using a calculator, solve for pH. Compare this calculated pH with the pH from the blood gas. If they match, the blood gas is internally consistent. If they don't match, an error has been made in reporting the blood gas. This check works because for given values of PCO$_2$ and [HCO$_3^-$], only one pH value is mathematically possible, and that value is defined by the H-H equation.

Patient 6. Interpret this ABG without knowing anything else about the patient.

ABG: pH = 7.40, $[HCO_3^-]$ = 18, PCO_2 = 30

Interpretation. This problem is a bit tricky because neither acidemia nor alkalemia is present, so you can't follow the usual 3-step sequence. Still, you should look at both $[HCO_3^-]$ and PCO_2, as you would normally. Both are low. For each of these variables, consider the possibility that the low level results from (1) the disturbance itself (primary change) or (2) the compensation (secondary change). There are three main possibilities to consider. First, a simple metabolic acidosis is present, with the low $[HCO_3^-]$ caused by the disturbance and the low PCO_2 caused by compensation (consistent with the same-direction rule; p. 55). However, compensation for metabolic disturbances does not bring pH into the normal range (p. 56), much less all the way to 7.4, so a simple metabolic acidosis is not possible. Second, a simple respiratory alkalosis is present, with the low PCO_2 caused by the disturbance and the low $[HCO_3^-]$ caused by the compensation (same-direction rule). Although compensation for respiratory alkalosis can bring pH into the normal range, it will not normally bring pH back to its set point value (i.e., the pre-disease starting point for the patient; pp. 59–60). Therefore, it is useful to know the patient's actual set point pH. If that information is not available to you from a previous lab report or chart record, assume that the set point pH is 7.4, the midpoint of the normal range. Based on this assumption, you can provisionally rule out compensated respiratory alkalosis.* Third, there is a mixed disturbance consisting of both metabolic acidosis and respiratory alkalosis, which have opposing (and canceling) effects on pH. This is the best choice. You have not definitively ruled out the second option (a well-compensated, simple respiratory alkalosis), but in the absence of other relevant information the mixed disturbance is your best working hypothesis.

Patient 6, continued. Reconsider the same patient, this time taking into account both the ABG and the following venous values:

$[Na^+]$ = 139, $[Cl^-]$ = 100, $[K^+]$ = 4.4, Total CO_2 = 17

Interpretation 6, continued. Calculate the anion gap. The elevated gap immediately suggests a gap metabolic acidosis, so a simple, chronic respiratory alkalosis is now ruled out. Since a simple metabolic acidosis cannot present with a normal pH, the disturbance must be mixed: a gap metabolic acidosis plus respiratory alkalosis.

Patient 7. A 16-year old male with a history of poorly controlled type 1 diabetes presents with these venous values: $[Na^+]$ = 142, $[Cl^-]$ = 97, $[K^+]$ = 3.6, Total CO_2 = 9, creatinine = 1.6, BUN = 27, glucose = 600 mg/dl. Plasma ketones are markedly elevated.

*****Going further.** Had pH been high-normal (say, 7.43) instead of 7.4, this might have been a well-compensated respiratory alkalosis. Alternatively, if you knew that this patient's normal set point was at the low end of the normal range (say, 7.36 or 7.37), a compensated pH of 7.4 would be possible, since this value is still slightly alkalemic relative to a low-normal set point.

The clinician had difficulty puncturing the artery and, unfortunately, several painful attempts were required. Eventually, the following ABG was obtained: pH = 7.38, [HCO_3^-] = 8, PCO_2 = 14. On physical exam, lungs are clear. Oxygen saturation by pulse oximetry is 99 percent. What is the likely diagnosis?

Interpretation. The very high plasma glucose, in conjunction with the low Total CO_2 and the elevated plasma ketone level, clearly points to diabetic ketoacidosis, especially given the history of type 1 diabetes. This diagnosis is consistent with the markedly elevated anion gap (36). However, the three-step analysis of the blood gas reveals that PCO_2 is below the expected compensatory range (rule p. 62, 130), indicating a superimposed respiratory alkalosis (i.e., there is a mixed disturbance: anion gap metabolic acidosis and respiratory alkalosis). Although you cannot definitively rule out respiratory disease from the information presented, the high oxygen saturation and clear lungs on physical exam reduce your suspicion for lung disease. A possibility you must take seriously—particularly since several arteriopuncture attempts were needed to obtain the blood sample—is that the patient developed an acute, transient respiratory alkalosis in response to pain and anxiety from arteriopuncture (p. 121).

Patient 8. A COPD patient with a history of hypercapnia presents with fever, cyanosis, and this blood gas: pH = 7.26, [HCO_3^-] = 30, PCO_2 = 70. The anion gap is normal. What is your thought process and what is the likely diagnosis?

Interpretation. In carrying out the three steps to interpret the blood gas, use the chronic respiratory acidosis rule (p. 63, 130) since the history indicates chronic hypercapnia. Using this rule, you see that [HCO_3^-] is lower than expected. Therefore, the respiratory acidosis is not fully compensated. Two main possibilities exist. The first possibility is that PCO_2 rose acutely from its already hypercapnic baseline due to an acute exacerbation of the COPD (acute-on-chronic respiratory acidosis p. 111, 122). Here, the assumption is that the prior, stable, chronic hypercapnia was fully compensated but the additional, acute rise in PCO_2 has not yet been present long enough for additional compensation (a further rise in [HCO_3^-]) to occur. The second possibility is that a metabolic acidosis, which reduced the [HCO_3^-], is superimposed on the chronic hypercapnia. Here, the assumption is that the hypercapnia is stable and that compensation was appropriate, but the metabolic acidosis reduced [HCO_3^-]. The patient's fever and cyanosis, which are consistent with an acute pulmonary infection, make the first possibility most likely. In contrast, if the patient had no new pulmonary symptoms but instead had diarrhea or some other potential cause of metabolic acidosis, you would have considered a superimposed metabolic acidosis. Cyanosis raises the possibility of lactic acidosis caused by hypoxemia (p. 71), but the normal anion gap points you away from this possibility. That said, a modest elevation in plasma lactate can sometimes "hide" within the normal range of the anion gap (e.g., if the baseline anion gap had been low-normal, lactate could rise several mmol/l without causing the anion gap to be above normal). A specific lactate assay could shed light on this possibility.

Patient 9. An acutely ill homeless woman with a history of alcoholism is brought to the emergency department in a stupor. What is the likely diagnosis?

Venous: $[Na^+]$ = 142, $[Cl^-]$ = 90, $[K^+]$ = 3.0, Total CO_2 = 10, Creatinine = 2.1, BUN = 28, glucose = 90.
ABG: pH = 7.33, $[HCO_3^-]$ = 9, PCO_2 = 24
Measured plasma osmolarity: 310 mOsm/l
Plasma ketones and lactate: negative
Urine ketones: positive

Interpretation. For the ABG, Steps 1–3 point to an appropriately compensated metabolic acidosis. The history and very high anion gap (42) raise the possibility of a toxic ingestion with methanol or ethylene glycol. The elevated creatinine, while by no means diagnostic, slightly raises your suspicion of ethylene glycol, because in ethylene glycol poisoning calcium oxalate crystals may deposit in the kidney and cause acute renal failure (pp. 77, 84); if renal failure is in its early stages, a creatinine around 2 is possible. The calculated plasma osmolarity is approximately 303, so the osmolar gap is only 7, which is within the normal range of –10 to +10 (p. 82). However, a normal osmolar gap does not rule out either methanol or ethylene glycol (p. 82). In fact, the very high anion gap suggests that much of the original ingestion has already been metabolized to toxic acids, thereby lowering the quantity of the neutral molecules (such as methanol and ethylene glycol), which is what is measured by the osmolar gap. Specific toxin assays should be sent to the lab. A urine sample should be examined for calcium oxalate crystals and tested with an ultraviolet light (p. 84) for the presence of fluorescent dye, which might suggest ingestion of ethylene-glycol containing auto antifreeze solution. Note that the elevated urine ketones in the presence of a normal plasma ketone level may suggest mild starvation ketoacidosis. (Since the urine ketone assay can be more sensitive than the plasma ketone assay, the combination of a negative plasma and positive urine assay may suggest low but undetectable plasma ketone levels.) Alcoholic ketoacidosis can sometimes present with a normal ketone test due to the test's insensitivity to beta-hydroxybutyrate (p. 80). Therefore, in this patient, you should request a specific beta-hydroxybutyrate assay, if one is available at your lab.

Patient 10. A debilitated, hospitalized patient on nasogastric drainage develops a fever. The patient's respiratory rate and depth increases, and blood pressure falls. Construct a plausible clinical scenario using these lab values:

Venous: $[Na^+]$ = 144, $[Cl^-]$ = 92, $[K^+]$ = 4.4, Total CO_2 = 27
ABG: pH = 7.56, $[HCO_3^-]$ = 26, PCO_2 = 30

Interpretation. The low PCO_2 and normal $[HCO_3^-]$ raise the possibility of an acute respiratory alkalosis, consistent with the increase in ventilation. (Hyperventilation, depending on its intensity, may or may not be observable, but when you do observe it, as in this patient, it is a helpful sign.) Given the onset of fever, perhaps the respiratory alkalosis indicates sepsis due to infection (p. 118). So at this point, as a working hypothesis, we can say that the patient probably has a more-or-less acute respiratory alkalosis. So far, so good—but this can't be the whole story because the anion gap is elevated, pointing to a gap metabolic acidosis. It is possible that this acidosis is a lactic acidosis from septic shock (p. 123, 71). A stat lactate assay would be helpful. So now, as the working hypothesis evolves, we have both an acute respiratory alkalosis and an anion gap metabolic acidosis—a mixed disturbance. Assuming that this metabolic acidosis is in fact present, you still need to explain why $[HCO_3^-]$ is not low, because normally a metabolic acidosis will cause $[HCO_3^-]$ to be low, whether or not acute respiratory alkalosis is also present. One possibility that can explain the normal $[HCO_3^-]$ is that the patient has a metabolic alkalosis from the nasogastric drainage (loss of gastric fluid, whether from vomiting or gastric drainage, is a common cause of metabolic alkalosis; pp. 94–96). So we're now considering the possibility that the patient had metabolic alkalosis, and that lactic acid from lactic acidosis consumed the excess bicarbonate, via buffering, thus bringing plasma $[HCO_3^-]$ to a normal level. (This "normal" $[HCO_3^-]$ level is merely the net result of two abnormal states, one tending to raise $[HCO_3^-]$ and the other tending to lower it.) That is, the patient may have first had a simple (not mixed) metabolic alkalosis, and then developed, in fairly close temporal sequence, both a respiratory alkalosis and metabolic acidosis. So now we're contemplating a *triple* mixed disturbance (metabolic alkalosis, acute respiratory alkalosis, and metabolic acidosis). That is our working diagnosis. Recall that metabolic alkalosis from nasogastric drainage (and also from vomiting and diuretics) are volume-responsive, meaning that they are associated with and maintained by volume depletion (p. 98). Thus, the patient may be volume depleted. This volume depletion may have contributed to the reduced tissue perfusion that underlies the lactic acidosis of septic shock (pp. 123, 71). So our hypothesis of a prior metabolic alkalosis makes sense in terms of the big picture, in that the associated volume depletion would increase the chance that the patient, once sepsis set in, would develop lactic acidosis. To recap: the scenario presented here is likely a triple mixed disturbance: metabolic alkalosis (nasogastric drainage), respiratory alkalosis (sepsis), and gap metabolic acidosis (septic shock)—probably arising in that order.

Congratulations! You've now completed the ten core problems in this chapter. To solve the final two problems, you'll need to think outside the box and figure out for yourself some relatively advanced concepts that are not covered in the main text. Challenge yourself—then check your conclusions. The interpretations will explain the new concepts.

Patient 11. ABG: pH = 7.33, $[HCO_3^-]$ = 22, PCO_2 = 43.
Is an acid-base disturbance present? If so, what is it?

Interpretation. In one sense, this problem is easy. Using Steps 1 & 2, you see that acidemia is present, and that the direction of this pH change can be accounted for by both PCO_2 and HCO_3^- (PCO_2 is higher than the mid-point of the normal range and $[HCO_3^-]$ is lower than the mid-point). This suggests that both respiratory acidosis and metabolic acidosis are present: a mixed disturbance. What is confusing is that even though pH is abnormal, both PCO_2 and HCO_3^- are themselves within the normal range. The resolution of this conundrum is that in a person *without* an acid-base disturbance, PCO_2 and HCO_3^- are not free to diverge one high and one low within the normal range, at least not far enough to cause pH to be abnormal. (Notice that, in the patient considered here, PCO_2 is high-normal and $[HCO_3^-]$ is low-normal—and it is this high-low combination that causes pH to be abnormal.) Instead, PCO_2 and HCO_3^- are always to some extent coordinated with each other, so as to keep pH in the normal range. For example, if PCO_2 is in the high-normal range, $[HCO_3^-]$ will tend to be in the high-normal range as well. (You can think of this situation as being consistent with the "same-direction" rule.) This coordination takes place because PCO_2 influences renal bicarbonate handling (a rise in PCO_2, even within the normal range, tends to slightly raise renal bicarbonate regeneration and reabsorption). Likewise, plasma $[HCO_3^-]$ tends to alter pulmonary function (a fall in $[HCO_3^-]$, even within the normal range, tends to increase ventilation). If this coordination is absent, resulting in an abnormal pH, you know that an acid-base disturbance is present, though it may be quite mild. So, in this problem, a mild, mixed disturbance (mild respiratory acidosis and mild metabolic acidosis) exists.

> **Patient 12.** Venous: $[Na^+]$ = 145, $[Cl^-]$ = 95, Total CO_2 = 20
> ABG: pH = 7.33, $[HCO_3^-]$ = 18, PCO_2 = 35
> There is something in these labs that hints at the presence of a mixed disturbance. What is it?

Interpretation. The low arterial $[HCO_3^-]$ and venous Total CO_2, in conjunction with the elevated anion gap, point to an anion gap metabolic acidosis. Using the Winters' formula, Step 3 of the blood gas analysis indicates that respiratory compensation is in the predicted range. So far, so good—but don't stop yet. Notice that the anion gap is 30, a truly marked elevation: if you assume a baseline gap of 12 (midpoint of the normal range), then the gap is elevated by 18 (30 – 12). However, the decrease in bicarbonate is fairly mild: assuming a starting value of 24, arterial $[HCO_3^-]$ is decreased by just 6 mmol/l. Thus, there is a striking disparity between the *increment* in the anion gap (18) and the *decrement* in bicarbonate (6). (You get the same 6 mmol/l decrement if you use venous values: a mid-normal TCO_2 of 26 minus the observed TCO_2 of 20.)

Under many circumstances, the anion gap will rise by about 1 unit (meq/l) for each 1 mmol/l decrease in $[HCO_3^-]$. This 1:1 relationship makes sense because, in metabolic acidosis, $[HCO_3^-]$ decreases as a result of buffering the acid. If that acid leaves an unmeasured anion behind (such as lactate or acetoacetate), you would expect the anion gap to rise by an amount equal to the fall in $[HCO_3^-]$. If we assume a 1:1 relationship, and presume that the anion gap rose by 18, we'd expect that plasma $[HCO_3^-]$ would be just 6 mmol/l (i.e., 24 – 18), much lower than what we actually observed. In reality, the 1:1 relationship is far from exact because many factors can influence both the anion gap and $[HCO_3^-]$. (For example, unmeasured anions may be excreted in the urine, lowering the gap; and some bicarbonate may shift out of cells and into the ECF, increasing plasma $[HCO_3^-]$.) However, these factors often tend to cancel each other, at least to some extent, bringing the result back towards 1:1. Therefore, the increment in the anion gap and the decrement in bicarbonate do not normally diverge as markedly as we observe in this patient.

How can you explain this large divergence? One important possibility is that an unrecognized bicarbonate-raising process (either metabolic alkalosis or the compensation for chronic respiratory acidosis) has kept $[HCO_3^-]$ from falling as much as it otherwise would have. So in this problem, we may well have a mixed disturbance consisting of an anion gap metabolic acidosis plus either a metabolic alkalosis or a chronic (compensated) respiratory acidosis. The take-home lesson here is that in patients with an anion gap metabolic acidosis, comparing the increment in the anion gap with the decrement in bicarbonate concentration can sometimes provide a clue that a mixed disturbance is present. This topic has many complexities, which go beyond the scope of this book, but I wanted to at least introduce you to it.*

---

*__Going further.__ If you set up a fraction, putting the increment of the anion gap (18) in the numerator and the decrement of $[HCO_3^-]$ (6) in the denominator, you get 18/6 or, simply, 3. Setting up this kind of fraction gives you a single, numerical measure of the relationship between the change in the anion gap and the change in the plasma $[HCO_3^-]$. This fraction has traditionally been called "delta/delta" (sometimes written Δ/Δ), which literally means "change/change" because the Greek letter delta (Δ) is used in math to indicate the change in a variable. However, I prefer to call the fraction by the more descriptive name "R/F," for Rise (in anion gap) over Fall (in bicarbonate), because this name reminds you how to set up the fraction. Using delta terminology can be doubly confusing because the term delta, and the symbol Δ, are sometimes used as synonyms for "anion gap"—that is, for the gap *itself*, as opposed to the *increment* in the gap. If you would like to learn more about this topic, as well as several other advanced topics related to the anion gap, you can download a free PDF titled "The Anion Gap: Taking It to the Next Level" at AcidBaseMadeClear.com.

Index

An "n" indicates footnote. When relevant information is found in both main text and footnote on same page, no "n" is given.

Made in the USA
Columbia, SC
14 August 2017